Public Health Surveillance

Public Health Surveillance

Edited by

William Halperin, M.D., M.P.H.
Edward L. Baker, Jr., M.D.

Consulting Editor

Richard R. Monson, M.D., Sc.D.

JOHN WILEY & SONS, INC.

New York • Chichester • Weinheim • Brisbane • Singapore • Toronto

Copyright © 1992 by John Wiley & Sons, Inc.
Originally published as ISBN 0-442-00762-0

For ordering and customer service, call 1-800-CALL-WILEY.

10 9 8 7 6 5 4 3 2

Library of Congress Cataloging-in-Publication Data
Public health surveillance / editors: William Halperin, Edward L.
 Baker ; consulting editor, Richard R. Monson.
     p. cm.
     "Compilation of essays . . . derive from lectures that were
 presented in a course at the Harvard School of Public Health in the
 fall of 1989"—Introd.
     Includes bibliographical references and index.
     1. Public health surveillance.
     [DNLM: 1. Population Surveillance—methods—essays. 2. Public
 Health—methods—essays. WA 105 P976]
 RA652.2.P82P83 1992
 614, 4—dc20
 DNLM/DLC   91-47926
 for Library of Congress   CIP

ISBN 0-471-28432-7

Contributors

EDWARD L. BAKER, M.D., M.P.H., M.Sc., Director, Public Health Practice Program Office, Centers for Disease Control, Atlanta, GA

RUTH L. BERKELMAN, M.D., Chief, Surveillance Branch, Division of HIV/AIDS, National Center for Infectious Diseases, Centers for Disease Control, Atlanta, GA

ROGER H. BERNIER, M.P.H., Ph.D., Chief, Epidemiology Research Section, Surveillance Investigations and Research Branch, Division of Immunization, National Center for Prevention Services, Centers for Disease Control, Atlanta, GA

STEPHEN B. BLOUNT, M.D., M.P.H. Director, Office of Surveillance and Analysis, National Center for Chronic Disease Prevention and Health Promotion, Centers for Disease Control, Atlanta, GA

JAMES W. BUEHLER, M.D., Chief, Special Projects Section, Division of HIV/AIDS, National Center for Infectious Diseases, Centers for Disease Control, Atlanta, GA

TIMOTHY J. DONDERO, JR., M.D., Chief, Seroepidemiology Branch, Division of HIV/AIDS, National Center for Infectious Diseases, Centers for Disease Control, Atlanta, GA

LARRY D. EDMONDS, M.S.P.H., Chief, Surveillance Section, Birth Defects and Genetic Diseases Branch, Division of Birth Defects and Developmental Disabilities, National Center for Environmental Health and Injury Control, Centers for Disease Control Public Health Service, U. S. Department of Health and Human Services, Atlanta, GA

TODD M. FRAZIER, Sc.M., Chief, Surveillance Branch, Division of Surveillance, Hazard Evaluations and Field Studies, National Institute for Occupational Safety and Health, Centers for Disease Control, Cincinnati, OH

v

PAUL L. GARBE, D.V.M., M.P.H., Chief, Chronic Disease Surveillance Branch, Office of Surveillance and Analysis, National Center for Health Promotion and Disease Prevention, Centers for Disease Control, Atlanta, GA

ROBERT P. GAYNES, M.D., Chief, Nosocomial Infections Surveillance Activity, Hospital Infections Program, National Center for Infectious Diseases, Centers for Disease Control, Atlanta, GA

ROGER I. GLASS, M.D., M.P.H., Ph.D., Chief, Viral Gastroenteritis Unit, Respiratory and Enterovirus Branch, Division of Viral and Rickettsial Diseases, National Center for Infectious Diseases, Centers for Disease Control, Atlanta, GA

PHILIP L. GRAITCER, D.M.D., M.P.H., Medical Epidemiologist, Division of Injury Control, National Center for Environmental Health and Injury Control, Centers for Disease Control, Atlanta, GA

WILLIAM HALPERIN, M.D., M.P.H., Associate Director for Surveillance, Division of Surveillance, Hazard Evaluations and Field Studies, National Institute for Occupational Safety and Health, Centers for Disease Control, Cincinnati, OH

GREGORY R. ISTRE, M.D., State Epidemiologist, Oklahoma State Department of Health, Oklahoma City, OK

DOUGLAS N. KLAUCKE, M.D., M.P.H., Director, Global Epidemic Intelligence Service, Epidemiology Program Office, Centers for Disease Control, Atlanta, GA

MICHELE C. LYNBERG, M.P.H., Ph.D., Medical Epidemiologist, Birth Defects and Genetic Diseases Branch, Division of Birth Defects and Developmental Disabilities, National Center for Environmental Health and Injury Control, Centers for Disease Control Public Health Service, U. S. Department of Health and Human Services, Atlanta, GA

MICHAEL D. MALISON, M.D., M.P.A., Deputy Director for Program, Global Epidemic Intelligence Service, Centers for Disease Control, Atlanta, GA

THOMAS P. MATTE, M.D., M.P.H., Medical Epidemiologist, Lead Poisoning Prevention Branch, Division of Environmental Hazards and Health Effects, National Center for Environmental Health and Injury Control, Centers for Disease Control, Atlanta, GA

RICHARD R. MONSON, M.D., Sc.D. Professor, Department of Epidemiology, School of Public Health, Harvard University, Boston, MA

ERIC K. NOJI, M.D., Assistant to the Branch Chief for Emergency Response, Health Studies Branch, Division of Environmental Hazards and Health Effects, National Center for Environmental Health and Injury Control, Centers for Disease Control, Atlanta, GA

WALTER A. ORENSTEIN, M.D., Director, Division of Immunization, National Center for Prevention Services, Centers for Disease Control, Atlanta, GA

PAUL J. SELIGMAN, M.D., M.P.H., Chief, Medical Section, Surveillance Branch, Division of Surveillance, Hazard Evaluations and Field Studies, National Institute for Occupational Safety and Health, Cincinnati, OH

STEPHEN B. THACKER, M.D., M.Sc., Director, Epidemiology Program Office, Centers for Disease Control, Atlanta, GA

HUGH H. TILSON, M.D., Dr.P.H., Director, Epidemiology, Surveillance and Pharmaco-economics Division, Burroughs Wellcome Company, Research Triangle Park, NC

DAVID H. WEGMAN, M.D., M.S., Professor and Chair, Department of Work Environment, College of Engineering, University of Massachusetts at Lowell, Lowell, MA

Contents

Preface

"Good surveillance does not necessarily ensure the making of the right decisions, but it reduces the chances of wrong ones."[1]

Public health surveillance is central to the process of disease prevention. Surveillance systems are vital tools in targeting the resources of the public health system and in evaluating program effectiveness. In *The Future of Public Health*,[2] the Institute of Medicine found the core functions of public health to be assessment, policy development, and assurance of the availability of services. Surveillance is intrinsic to the assessment function and esssential for proper policy development and assurance of service availability.

Modern disease prevention and health promotion programs require meaningful data systems if the Unitess States is to achieve the Year 2000 National Health Promotion and Disease Prevention Objectives. As an indication of their importance, a separate set of Year 2000 Health Objectives were developed to focus attention on surveillance and data systems. One of the most important is the development of a uniform set of health indicators to be used by all federal, state, and local agencies to monitor progress (Objective 22:1).[3]

This book is designed to address an ongoing national dialogue on the role of public health education in training future public health professionals; graduates of schools of public health are acknowledging the need for more books and course materials designed to prepare students for public health practice. State and local public health agencies in particular have recognized this need as they recruit and hire new professional staff.

We hope that this book will provide a useful tool to faculty schools of public health as they design and conduct courses on public health surveillance.

Many deserve thanks for their role in creating this book. The origin of the book is a course on the subject organized by one of us (WH) given at the Harvard School of Public Health in 1989. Without the essential guidance of Richard Monson, the advice of Ian Greaves of the University of Minnesota, and the assistance of Arthur Liang of the Centers for Disease Control, that course and this book would never have become reality. A talented group of students also offered valuable advice on the content of this book. Those who contributed chapters deserve the greatest thanks. We were extremely fortunate in obtaining the very best U.S. experts in a variety of surveillance areas; we and those who read this book are indebted to them. The staff and editors who helped to assemble this book labored diligently and deserve the highest praise, especially Juanita Nelson, who converted the contributed chapters into a common format and word processing language. Immeasurable appreciation must be expressed to those epidemiologists who have made surveillance an essential component of the practice of public health, particularly Alexander Langmuir. We all hope that our efforts will serve to advance the mission of public health—"to fulfill society's interest in assuring conditions in which people can be healthy."

Notes
1. Langmuir A. D. 1963. The surveillance of communicable diseases of national importance. *NEJM* 268:182–192.
2. Institute of Medicine. 1988. *The Future of Public Health*. Washington, D.C.: National Academy Press.
3. Public Health Service. 1991. *Healthy People 2000; National Health Promotion and Disease Prevention Objectives*. Washington, D.C.: U.S. Department of Health and Human Services.

Introduction

William Halperin

This book is a compilation of essays on the role of surveillance in the prevention of disease and injury which derive from lectures that were presented in a course at the Harvard School of Public Health in the fall of 1989. Although surveillance is an essential element of the practice of public health, the subject is rarely taught in schools of public health or fully discussed in textbooks on public health or epidemiology. This gap reflects the disjunction between schools of public health and public health practitioners recently addressed in a report by the Institute of Medicine, *The Future of Public Health.*[1] It is our hope that this book will help to bridge this widening gap.

This book parallels the design of the course, both were designed for introductory students. The course began with a series of prefatory lectures on such broad issues as the history of surveillance, and the evaluation of surveillance programs, and continued with more narrowly focused lectures that demonstrated the use of surveillance, particularly the modification of general surveillance concepts, in the prevention of specific diseases such as the vaccine preventable diseases and HIV/AIDS. Focusing on basic principles, the chapters provide a limited number of references for readers seeking a starting point to explore the relevant literature, though they are not meant to provide an exhaustive review.

This book cannot reproduce the field experience component of the course. Students identified surveillance programs in the Boston area, and in small groups visited the program in order to understand its purpose, functions, limitations, and so forth. The students then evaluated the surveillance program using the principles presented in this volume, and reviewed their findings with the class. We recommend that courses using this book require similar field experiences, using the book to provide a framework for a practical, problem-oriented approach to solving problems of public health importance.

The course began (as does this book) with a discussion of the differences among epidemiology, surveillance, and public health. Surveillance, as defined by Alexander Langmuir, "means the continued watchfulness over the distribution and trends of incidence through the systematic collection, consolidation and evaluation of morbidity and mortality reports and other relevant data"[2,3] for the purposes of prevention of disease or injury. Other modifications of this definition are discussed throughout the book. However, it is worth lingering now over some of the key words in this version of the definition. Notice that "continued watchfulness" implies that the surveillance process continues over time, rather than being a one-time survey or epidemiologic study. Repeated surveys from which trends can be discerned are consistent with surveillance. "Collection, consolidation, and evaluation" should differentiate surveillance as a process from the equally important but different enterprise of registering cases in a disease register. "Other relevant data" allows for collection of information on risk factors for disease, health or safety hazards, or preventive interventions, such as immunization, rather than limiting surveillance to the collection of data solely on disease. To differentiate surveillance from other useful collection of data (such as marketing surveys for a product), "for the purposes of prevention of injury and disease," has been added to Dr. Langmuir's definition. Surveillance should not be so rigidly defined that in-depth investigations of individual or sentinel cases representing a failure of prevention, such as a maternal death or an industrial injury, are excluded.

Public health is defined as the logical application of methods of problem recognition, evaluation, and intervention for the prevention of disease and injury in populations. A working definition of epidemiology should reflect both the traditional, broad notion that epidemiology is "the study of the distribution and determinants of disease frequency in man,"[4] which encompasses interest in epidemic and endemic diseases as well as an alternate view of theoretical epidemiology. Theoretical of modern epidemiology focuses much more on the use of very sophisticated analytic methodology for understanding the relationship of risk factor and disease, particularly of endemic disease, rather than on the description of epidemics.[5]

A useful model for the presentation of the role of surveillance in the practice of public health has been developed by Greenwald,[6] further elaborated by Layde,[7] and modified here. The first step in public health is the recognition of a problem. Surveillance can be used to identify an upward trend in cases of a known disease such as measles, or to recognize a new disease, such as in the first reports of toxic shock syndrome by physicians to public health agencies.

The second step in public health is the definition of the scope of a problem. For example, the collection and analysis of laboratory reports of elevated lead levels in adults, and subsequent followup with these adults, can be used to estimate the prevalence of occupational lead poisoning in the United States. The ongoing collection, analysis, and use of these laboratory reports for the purpose of prevention is an example of surveillance and part of the public health process for eliminating lead poisoning.

The third step in the public health process is to conduct etiologic research to determine the cause of a disease. This step consists of an epidemiologic study, not surveillance. For example, an epidemiologic study might be conducted to determine the differential exposure of cases of eosinophilia-myalgia syndrome as compared to controls without the disease. It does not require the ongoing collection of information about cases, but only about cases occurring during the research period.

Once an etiologic agent or exposure is identified, the next step in the public health process is the design of an intervention that will prevent transmission of the infectious agent, exposure to a chemical hazard, and so forth. Examples of intervention include immunization, withdrawal of a food contaminant, or repair of a ventilation system. This is not surveillance. Once an intervention is developed, it must be tried in an experimental situation to determine if it is effective. This type of public health experiment is also not an example of surveillance.

If the intervention is effective in the experimental situation, the targeting of the intervention should be guided by surveillance information that identifies high-risk groups. For example, success in the eradication of smallpox was accomplished by conducting intensive surveillance for cases and targeting immunization to the contacts of cases. Similarly, greater success in cancer prevention may be accomplished if screening programs for breast cancer and cervical cancer were targeted to high-risk populations.

Finally, surveillance is useful in evaluating the effectiveness of a public health intervention by assessing the trend in disease or injury once the intervention becomes a routine component of public health programs. For example, surveillance of roll-over fatalities from farm tractors in Sweden[8] demonstrated some decline after a requirement in 1958 that all new tractors have roll bars. However, the incidence of roll-over fatalities did not substantially subside until 1978, when a new law mandated that all tractors in use must have roll-over protection. Alternately, surveillance is of value in tracking the use of the preventive intervention; for example, the number and demographic characteristics of children who are not immunized.

The definitions and model of public health presented here should serve to differentiate surveillance from the whole of public health practice, and to distinguish surveillance from analytic epidemiologic studies. These issues will reappear with substantially more discussion in subsequent chapters and should provide an adequate foundation for exploring the questions posed in remainder of this volume.

Notes
1. Institute of Medicine. 1988. *The Future of Public Health*. Washington, D.C.: National Academy Press.
2. Langmuir, A. D. 1963. The surveillance of communicable diseases of national importance. *NEJM* 268:182–191.
3. Langmuir, A. D. 1976. William Farr: founder of modern concepts of surveillance. *Int J Epidemiol* 5:13–18.
4. MacMahon, B. and T. Pugh. 1970. *Epidemiology: Principles and Methods*. Boston; Little, Brown and Company.
5. Miettinen, O. 1985. *Theoretical Epidemiology: Principles of Occurrence Research in Medicine*. New York: John Wiley and Sons.
6. Greenwald, P., J. W. Cullen, and J. W. McKenna. 1987. Cancer prevention and control: from research through application. *JNCI* 79:389–400.
7. Layde, P. 1990. Beyond surveillance: methodologic considerations in analytic studies of agricultural injuries. *Am J Ind Med* 18:193–200.
8. Thelin, A. 1990. Epilogue: agricultural, occupational, and environmental health policy strategies for the future. *Am J Ind Med* 18:523–526.

Public Health Surveillance

1

History of Public Health Surveillance

Stephen B. Thacker and Ruth L. Berkelman

The Centers for Disease Control (CDC) defines public health surveillance as

> the ongoing, systematic collection, analysis, and interpretation of health data
> essential to the planning, implementation, and evaluation of public health
> practice, closely integrated with the timely dissemination of these data to those
> who need to know. The final link of the surveillance chain is the application of
> these data to prevention and control. A surveillance system includes a functional
> capacity for data collection, analysis, and dissemination linked to public health
> programs.[1]

In this chapter, we trace the evolution of this concept from ancient and
medieval times; describe its role in the world's greatest public health
success, the eradication of smallpox; and illustrate the application of
public health surveillance to today's major public health concerns, such as
chronic disease, injury, and environmental health.

The process of observing, recording, and collecting facts and the analysis of the direct courses of medical intervention dates from the time of
Hippocrates.[2] The first real public health action that can be related to
surveillance probably occurred in 1348 during the bubonic plague, when
public health authorities boarded ships in the port near the Republic of
Venice to prevent persons suffering from a plague-like illness from disem-
barking.[3] Before an organized system of surveillance could be developed,
however, certain prerequisites needed to be met. First, there had to be
some semblance of an organized health care system in a stable government; this was not achieved until the time of the Roman Empire. Second,
a classification system for disease and illness had to be established and

accepted; this did not begin until the seventeenth century, with the work of Sydenham. Finally, mathematical methods for sophisticated statistical measurement had also not been developed until that time.

Current concepts of public health surveillance evolve from public health activities developed to control and prevent disease in the community. In the late Middle Ages, governments in Western Europe assumed responsibility for health protection and health care of the population of their towns and cities.[4] A rudimentary system of monitoring illness led to regulations against polluting streets and public water, instructions for burial and food handling, and the provision of some types of health care.[5]

In the 1680s, von Leibnitz called for the establishment of a health council and the application of a numerical analysis in mortality statistics to health planning. About the same time in London, John Graunt published a book, *Natural and Political Observations Made upon the Bills of Mortality,* in which he attempted to define the basic laws of natality and mortality. In his work, Graunt developed some fundamental principles of public health surveillance, including disease-specific death counts, death rates, and the concept of disease patterns. In the next century, Achenwall introduced the term "statistics," and over the next several decades the use of vital statistics became more widely spread in Europe. In 1766, Johann Peter Frank advocated a more comprehensive form of public health surveillance with the system of police medicine in Germany. It covered school health, injury prevention, maternal and child health, and public water and sewage, in addition to delineating governmental measures to protect the public health.[4] Nearly a century later, in 1845, Thurnam published the first extensive report of mental health statistics in London.

Two prominent names in the history of public health surveillance activities are Lemuel Shattuck and William Farr. Shattuck's 1850 report of the Massachusetts Sanitary Commission was a landmark publication that related death, infant and maternal mortality, and communicable diseases to living conditions. Shattuck also proposed a standardization of nomenclature for the causes of disease and death, and the collection of health data by age, sex, occupation, socioeconomic level, and locality. He applied these concepts to program activities in immunization, school health, smoking, and alcohol abuse, and introduced these concepts into the teaching of preventive medicine. William Farr (1807–1883) formulated the basic principles of surveillance.[6, 7] As superintendent of the statistical department of the Registrar General's office of England and Wales from 1839 to 1879, Farr concentrated his efforts on collecting vital statistics, on assembling and evaluating those data, and on reporting his results to both the responsible authorities and to the general public.

In the United States, public health surveillance has focused primarily upon infectious diseases. Basic elements of surveillance were present in Rhode Island in 1741 when the colony passed an act requiring tavern keepers to report contagious disease among their patrons. Two years later, the colony passed a law requiring the reporting of smallpox, yellow fever, and cholera.[8] National disease-monitoring activities did not begin until 1850, when mortality statistics based on the decennial census were first published by the federal government for the entire United States.[9] Systematic disease reporting in the United States began in 1874 when the Massachusetts State Board of Health instituted a voluntary plan for weekly reporting of prevalent diseases by physicians,[10] using a standard postcard reporting format.[11] In comparison, for example, compulsory reporting of infectious diseases began in Italy in 1881 and Great Britain in 1899. In 1878, Congress authorized the forerunner of the Public Health Service (PHS) to collect morbidity data for its use in quarantine measures against pestilential diseases such as cholera, smallpox, plague, and yellow fever.[12] In 1893, Michigan became the first U.S. jurisdiction to require the reporting of specific infectious diseases. In 1893, an act provided for the collection of information each week from state and municipal authorities throughout the United States. By 1901, all state and municipal laws required the notification of local authorities (i.e., reporting) of selected communicable diseases such as smallpox, tuberculosis, and cholera.[13] In 1914, PHS personnel were appointed as collaborating epidemiologists to serve in state health departments to telegraph reports weekly to the PHS.

It was not until 1925, however, following markedly increased reporting associated with the severe poliomyelitis epidemic in 1916 and the influenza pandemic in 1918 to 1919, that all states began participating in national morbidity reporting.[14] A national health survey of U.S. citizens was first conducted in 1935 by the National Office of Vital Statistics. After a 1948 PHS study led to the revision of morbidity reporting procedures, the National Office of Vital Statistics assumed the responsibilities for morbidity reporting. In 1949, weekly morbidity statistics that had appeared for several years in *Public Health Reports* were published by the National Office of Vital Statistics. In 1952, mortality data were added to what is now known as the *Morbidity and Mortality Weekly Report (MMWR)*. Since 1961, this publication has been the responsibility of the CDC.

The post–World War II malaria experience in the United States emphasized the necessity of a more current and comprehensive system of surveillance. The Malaria Eradication Program was undertaken by the CDC and state health departments in 1946 to address endemic malaria in the United States at a time when World War II veterans were returning from the African, Mediterranean, and Pacific theaters and introducing *Plasmodium vivax* to the population.[6] Spraying of dichlorodiphenyltrichloroethane

(DDT) had begun before surveillance was initiated. By 1947, it was clear that earlier reports of morbidity and mortality had been erroneous. Mississippi, South Carolina, and Texas had the highest reported incidences of malaria, but because there was no diagnostic verification, the rate of occurrence was exaggerated. A change in reporting requirements that included case reports with diagnostic clarification was illuminating. In Mississippi, for example, the incidence dropped from 17,764 to 914 reported cases in the first year—only a few of which could be confirmed. Such new criteria revealed that malaria had disappeared as an endemic disease from the South.

The critical demonstration in the United States of the importance of surveillance was made following the Francis Field Trial of poliomyelitis vaccine in 1955.[15, 16] Within two weeks of the announcement of the results of the field trial and the initiation of a nationwide vaccination program, six cases of paralytic poliomyelitis were reported through the notifiable disease reporting system to state and local health departments; case investigations revealed that these children had received vaccine made by a single manufacturer. The surgeon general requested that this manufacturer recall all outstanding lots of the vaccine and directed that a national poliomyelitis program be established at the CDC. Intensive surveillance and appropriate epidemiologic investigations by federal, state, and local health departments found 141 vaccine-associated cases of paralytic diseases, 80 of which involved family contacts. Daily surveillance reports were distributed by the CDC to all persons involved in these investigations. This national common-source epidemic was ultimately related to a particular brand of vaccine that had been contaminated with live virus. Had the surveillance program not been in existence, many and perhaps all vaccine manufacturers would have ceased production.

In the United States, the authority to require the notification of cases of disease within a state resides in the appropriate state legislature. In some states, authority is enumerated in statutory provisions; in others, the authority to require reporting has been given to state boards of health; still other states require reports under both statutes and health department regulations. State reporting requirements also vary among conditions and diseases to be reported, time frames for reporting, agencies receiving reports, persons required to report, conditions under which reports are required, and penalties for not reporting.[17]

The Conference (now Council) of State and Territorial Epidemiologists (CSTE) was authorized in 1951 by its parent body, the Association of State and Territorial Health Officials, to determine what diseases should be reported by states to the PHS and to develop reporting procedures. The Council currently meets annually and—in collaboration with the

CDC—recommends to its constituents appropriate changes in morbidity reporting and surveillance, including what diseases should be reported to the CDC and published in the *MMWR*.

Until 1950, the term "surveillance" was restricted in public health practice to watching contacts of serious communicable diseases such as smallpox, to detect early symptoms so that prompt isolation could be instituted.[18] Formulation of the modern concept of public health surveillance has generally been attributed to Alexander D. Langmuir. In 1963, Langmuir defined disease surveillance as the "continued watchfulness over the distribution and trends of incidence through the systematic collection, consolidation, and evaluation of morbidity and mortality reports and other relevant data," and the regular dissemination to "all who need to know."[6] Langmuir was careful to distinguish surveillance both from direct responsibility for control activities and from epidemiologic research, although he recognized the important interplay among epidemiologic studies, surveillance, and control activities.

In May 1966, the Nineteenth World Health Assembly decided to initiate a program for the global eradication of smallpox under the auspices of the World Health Organization. The program was begun in 1967 with a 10-year plan based on a coordinated campaign of mass vaccination, assessment, surveillance, and maintenance activities. The critical strategic element that enabled successful attainment of the program goal was the implementation in 1968 of a surveillance-containment strategy that included active surveillance of all cases of smallpox during seasonal periods of low incidence and aggressive vaccination around these cases. D. A. Henderson has said, "Ultimately a single element, a single addition to the strategy of the [eradication] program was responsible [for its success]—that change was the incorporation of the principle of surveillance."[19]

In 1968 the Twenty-first World Health Assembly focused on the national and global surveillance of communicable diseases, applying the term to diseases rather than to the monitoring of individuals with selected communicable diseases.[20] At that assembly, it was confirmed that surveillance required (1) the systematic collection of pertinent data, (2) the orderly consolidation and evaluation of these data, and (3) the prompt dissemination of results to those who need to know, particularly those in a position to take action. Since then, a wide variety of health events—such as childhood lead poisoning, leukemia, congenital malformations, abortions, injuries, and behavioral risk factors—have been brought under surveillance. In 1976, recognition of the breadth of surveillance activities throughout the world was made evident by a special issue of the *International Journal of Epidemiology* devoted to health surveillance.[21]

Surveillance has assumed major significance in disease control and prevention. Its specific connotations, however, have not been universally understood. In 1963, Langmuir clearly limited surveillance to the collection, analysis, and dissemination of data.[6] The term did not encompass direct responsibility for control activities. In 1965, the director general of the World Health Organization (WHO) established the epidemiologic surveillance unit in the Division of Communicable Diseases of WHO.[22] The division director, Karel Raska, defined surveillance much more broadly than Langmuir, and included in his definition "the epidemiological study of disease as a dynamic process." In the case of malaria, he saw epidemiologic surveillance as encompassing control and prevention activities. Indeed, the WHO definition of malaria surveillance included not only case detection but also blood films, drug treatment, epidemiologic investigation, and follow-up.[23]

The 1968 World Health Assembly discussions reflected the broadened concepts of epidemiologic surveillance and addressed the application of the concept to public health problems other than communicable diseases.[20] In addition, epidemiologic surveillance was said to imply "the responsibility of following up to see that effective action has been taken."

The application of the term "epidemiologic" to surveillance first appeared in the mid-1960s, and was associated with the establishment of the WHO unit of that name. This was done to distinguish this activity from other forms of surveillance, such as military intelligence, and to reflect its broader applications. The use of the term "epidemiologic," however, engenders both confusion and controversy. In 1971, Langmuir noted that some epidemiologists tended to equate surveillance with epidemiology in its broadest sense, including epidemiologic investigations and research.[18] He found this "both epidemiologically and administratively unwise," favoring a definition of surveillance as "epidemiological intelligence."

What are the boundaries of surveillance practice? Is "epidemiologic" an appropriate modifier of "surveillance" as the terms are used in public health practice? To address these questions, we must first examine the structure of public health practice. One can divide public health activities into surveillance, epidemiologic and laboratory research, service (including program evaluation), and training. Surveillance data should be used to identify areas needed in research and service, that, in turn, help to define training needs. Unless these data are provided to those who set policy and implement programs, their use is limited to archival and academic pursuits, and are appropriately considered to be health information rather than surveillance data. Though both may be based on surveillance, they are independent public health activities. Hence, the boundary of surveillance practice is drawn before the actual conduct of research and the implementation of delivery programs.

Given this context, using "epidemiologic" as a modifier for "surveillance" is misleading. Epidemiology is a broad discipline that incorporates research and training that is distinct from a public health process we call surveillance. Because of the much broader content of epidemiology, the use of "epidemiologic" confuses the meaning of surveillance in the public health setting, having led in the past to the inappropriate incorporation of research into the definition of surveillance.[23] The term "public health surveillance" retains the original benefits of the term "epidemiologic" cited previously and removes the confusion surrounding current practice. Surveillance is more correctly an element of public health, and persons encountering this term should understand this.

APPLICATION OF PROGRAM

The concept of public health surveillance has evolved from a primarily archival function prior to 1950 to one in which there is timely analysis of the data with an appropriate response. Because surveillance is part of public health practice, it should be used for guiding control and/or prevention measures (or relevant research). No public health surveillance system is complete without being linked to action. The uses of surveillance include detecting new health problems (e.g., antibiotic-resistant strains of bacteria), detecting epidemics, documenting the spread of disease, providing quantitative estimates of the magnitude of morbidity and mortality, describing the clinical course of disease, identifying potential factors involved in disease occurrence, facilitating epidemiologic research, targeting resources for program intervention, and assessing contol of prevention activities.

Surveillance activities, however, have frequently led to epidemiologic investigations of etiology. After the initiation of the National Influenza Immunization Program in October 1976, cases of Guillain-Barré syndrome were reported to the CDC through a nationwide surveillance system established to monitor illnesses associated with influenza vaccination.[24] Subsequent epidemiologic studies demonstrated a relationship between Guillain-Barré syndrome and the swine influenza vaccine that was in use, which resulted in the cessation of the vaccination program for the year.[25] To test whether the syndrome could result from the use of other influenza vaccines, a special surveillance system was established in 1978 that enlisted 1,813 neurologists as reporters.[26] The data collected for that year and several subsequent years showed no association between the other influenza vaccines and Guillain-Barré syndrome.

In addition, public health surveillance systems are often the sources for case-control studies. For example, in response to concerns expressed by

Vietnam veterans about the possibility of increased risk for fathering children born with birth defects, the CDC conducted a case-control study using cases with serious structural birth defects identified by the Metropolitan Atlanta Congenital Defects Program.[27] The surveillance system attempted to ascertain all infants with defects diagnosed during the first year of life or born to mothers who resided in the area. Cases and controls were selected from infants born alive in the Atlanta area in the period 1968 to 1980. This study found that Vietnam veterans did not have an increased risk of fathering children with defects. Other examples of epidemiologic research facilitated by case ascertainment through surveillance included the demonstration of the association of tampon use with the development of toxic shock syndrome,[28] the relationship between salicylate use and Reye syndrome,[29] the risk of breast cancer associated with long-term oral contraceptive use,[30] and quantification of the risk of acquired immunodeficiency syndrome (AIDS) from certain sexual practices.[31]

Public health surveillance efforts have often been intensified when the means for primary prevention of most or all cases is at hand (e.g., vaccine for measles or smallpox) or when the disease is severe and newly emerging, with major efforts being made to develop control and prevention measures (e.g., toxic shock syndrome in the early 1980s). Additionally, public health surveillance has served as the means of identifying persons with the relevant health problem who can participate in epidemiologic studies for developing prevention strategies. Even before AIDS was documented as having a viral etiology, for example, measures to lower the risk for disease were suggested by cases detected through public health surveillance.[31]

NEW PUBLIC HEALTH PRIORITIES

The concepts of public health surveillance that have evolved from the prevention and control activities for acute infectious diseases are now being applied to such new areas of public health as chronic diseases, occupational safety and health, environmental health, injuries, personal health practices, and preventive health technologies.[32]

There has been extensive experience in data collection for the analysis of chronic disease occurrence, such as in population-based community studies of stroke and cardiovascular disease and community-based registries of hypertension and cancer. None of these data-collection activities, however, constitutes a public health surveillance system. The usefulness of existing data sets for chronic disease surveillance has not been proven, and to date there has been relatively little effort to apply the principles of public health surveillance to specific chronic conditions or to assess alternate approaches to collecting chronic disease data for public health surveillance. There are difficulties, however, in developing systems of public health surveillance for chronic disease. First, for some diseases that involve a one-time, discrete exposure (e.g., mesothelioma following asbestos exposure), the long latency period between the precipitating event or exposure and the eventual chronic disease not only hinders linkage but also complicates the development and evaluation of prevention programs. Second, the multifactorial etiology of many chronic conditions often prevents accurate linkage of exposures, risk factors, interventions, and outcomes. Third, because the public health community is often interested in reversing the progression of the chronic condition, surveillance at a number of stages of disease is important. For example, one would want to track both Stage I cervical cancer and mortality from cervical cancer. These difficulties should not, however, deter public health professionals from initiating chronic disease surveillance systems, because such surveillance has been shown to be useful in the detection of epidemics and in evaluating the effectiveness of primary and secondary prevention measures.[33]

Major efforts are under way to perform surveillance of occupational disease at both the national and state levels.[34] A survey conducted by the Iowa Department of Health in 1985 and 1986 showed that at least 30 states (60 percent) had either voluntary or mandatory reporting programs for selected occupational health conditions.[35] The states have not been uniform, however, in their reporting criteria for these occupational health events. Reporting to health departments will be expanded through the Sentinel Event Notification System for Occupational Risks (SENSOR), a health reporting system based on reporting selected occupational disease and injury outcomes amenable to control and prevention.[34]

Public health surveillance in environmental health includes both hazard (exposure) and health-effects monitoring. The most extensive public health surveillance system developed for an environmental hazard evolved from 62 childhood lead poisoning prevention programs.[36] Over a 10-year period (ending in 1981), 247,000 children with elevated lead levels were identified among nearly 4 million screened. When federal funding was discontinued in 1981, the national program stopped, and most local activities were curtailed or eliminated. Probably the most firmly established public health surveillance system related to environmental outcomes is that established for the surveillance of congenital malformations. The Metropolitan Atlanta Congenital Defects Program and the nationwide Birth Defects Monitoring Program, established in 1967 and 1974 respectively, made possible the monitoring of trends of specific birth defects or combinations of defects and have stimulated epidemiologic investigation to identify teratogens in the environment.[37] The primary challenge in the public health surveillance of environmental hazards is determining which hazards warrant ongoing programs of surveillance. The major constraint of the outcome approach is the limited knowledge of the health effects of specific toxins (i.e., natural) and toxicants (i.e., human-made) that inhibits our ability to detect unexpected associations between disease and exposure. Once priorities are established, data must be identified for both exposures and outcome, using—one would hope—already existing data sets.

The recognition of both intentional (e.g., homicide) and unintentional (e.g., falls) injuries as major health problems has led to the need for developing systems of public health surveillance for injuries.[38] Because of the acute nature of injury events, principles learned from experience with acute infectious diseases are often readily adaptable to injuries.[39] Approaches to surveillance for injuries vary at the state and local levels. In 1987, the CSTE adopted a resolution to recommend that spinal cord injury be made reportable in all states.[40] Trauma registries can also be adapted to surveillance. Several national data sets are available for the surveillance of unintentional injuries, such as those compiled at the National Center for Health Statistics of CDC, which collects and analyzes mortality statistics, hospital discharge data, office-based physician utilization data, and data collected in an ongoing health interview survey of the general population. As with chronic diseases, the usefulness of many of these data sources for public health surveillance needs to be assessed.

Intentional injuries are even more complex. Data are available from vital records and medical examiners, but information about the circumstances of homicide and suicide is often absent or limited in these data sets. Public health surveillance of intentional injuries will require the collaboration of the public health community with a different array of experts, including those in the fields of law enforcement and sociology.[41] Current efforts in the surveillance of suicide have demonstrated the importance and difficulty of arriving at uniform definitions, a problem complicated by the interdisciplinary nature of this endeavor. Nevertheless, as such databases are developed, surveillance will play a crucial role in public health programs aimed at controlling and preventing these and other injuries. Surveillance of personal health practices such as alcohol use and smoking is available through the National Health Interview Survey conducted by the CDC, as well as state and local data collected through the Behavioral Risk Factor Surveillance System.[42, 43] Results of these surveys are published both by the CDC and state health departments and distributed to the press and a variety of local and state organizations, including voluntary health agencies, hospitals, health maintenance organizations, and state legislatures. There are limitations on these survey data, but they do provide useful information for public health program planning and evaluation.

The surveillance of health technologies such as drugs, devices, and medical and surgical procedures used in health care is quite rudimentary. Vaccination against selected infectious diseases is probably the most effective and well-known technology used in public health. The implementation of new technology such as carotid endarterectomy, artificial hearts, and osteoporosis screening generally lacks useful systems of public health surveillance. Concerns regarding premature diffusion and misapplication of such technologies have highlighted the need for routine surveillance, particularly as these new technologies are used to prevent disease in healthy, asymptomatic populations.[44] The public health surveillance of new technologies provides a mechanism for monitoring the use of a practice or device and, together with data on related morbidity and mortality, provides an ongoing measure of its effectiveness and safety in the populations being monitored. Surveillance will also indicate whether effective technologies are being applied to the population that is most likely to benefit from such technology. The process of gathering primary data for surveillance is not established for most technologies; drugs are the responsibility of the Food and Drug Administration.[45] Although surveillance is usually undertaken by public health agencies at the local, state, and federal levels in collaboration with the medical community, efforts to establish surveillance systems at all levels have faltered in the area of preventive health technologies. Recently, the Behavioral Risk Factor Surveillance System has collected data in selected states on screening for cancer of the breast, cervix, or colon.

NEW TOOLS FOR PUBLIC HEALTH SURVEILLANCE

The replacement of pencil and paper with computer hardware and software has provided the public health professional with the capability to perform surveillance more efficiently on common conditions. Large databases may be better managed and analyzed, and in some instances may be linked. In addition, the microcomputer has empowered the public health professional with an increased ability to organize, communicate, tabulate, and analyze data. Use of the computer has improved the timeliness of both data collection and analysis and has decreased the epidemiologist's reliance on programmers and biostatisticians for data analysis and interpretation.

The usefulness of sentinel physician practices for surveillance has been demonstrated in the United Kingdom,[46] Belgium,[47] and other European countries. In France, a computerized, physician-based network has been implemented for national public health surveillance.[48] As of 1989, all state health departments in the United States are communicating notifiable disease data each week to the CDC through the National Electronic Tele-communication Surveillance System (NETSS). In addition, states have initiated computer linkage with selected local health departments for disease reporting.[49] The use of microcomputers has also expanded surveillance activities to nontraditional reporting sources such as medical examiners' offices and hospitals. Various sophisticated statistical methods have been made accessible by computerization. As a consequence, the usefulness of time series analysis,[50] of detecting clusters of adverse health events in time and place,[51] and of mathematical models to forecast epidemics based on surveillance data[52] is being assessed.

CONCLUSIONS

Public health surveillance provides a quantitative basis both for epidemiologic research and for control and prevention services. Public health surveillance includes not only data collection and analysis, but also the application of these data to control and prevention activities by disseminating information to practitioners of public health and to others who need to know. Although surveillance has been conducted in some form for more than a century, its uses and practices have evolved most dramatically over the past 40 years. One significant change has been the extension of surveillance beyond infectious disease to include the spectrum of public health problems of chronic disease, occupational health, injury, the environment, personal behavior, and preventive health technologies. Another significant change has been the effort to conduct public health surveillance on a more scientific basis, which will facilitate more effective use of surveillance data.[53]

Public health surveillance has been recognized as an early warning system, a crude indication of the occurrence of unusual disease patterns. Because of the focus on timeliness and simplicity, there has often been less concern for data quality. In recent years, however, there has been an increased use of data obtained outside of public health practice and an attendant, increasing concern for the quality of surveillance data and the methods used to collect and analyze these data.[54] It is appropriate, therefore, to examine and to ascertain how one can efficiently improve the collection, analysis, and dissemination of surveillance data.

The critical challenge in public health surveillance today, however, continues to be the assurance of its usefulness. For this purpose, we need rigorous evaluation of public health surveillance systems. Even more basic is the need to regard surveillance as a scientific endeavor. To do this properly, one must fully understand the principles of surveillance and its role in epidemiologic research and other aspects of the overall mission of public health. What is necessary is to develop epidemiologic methods relevant to public health surveillance; to apply computer technology for efficient data collection, analysis, and graphic display; to apply surveillance principles to new areas of public health practice; and to routinely reassess the usefulness of the surveillance systems.

Notes

1. Centers for Disease Control. January 1988. *CDC Surveillance Update*. Atlanta, Ga.: CDC.
2. Eylenbosch, W. J., and N. D. Noah. 1988. Historical aspects. In: *Surveillance in Health and Disease*, 3–8. Oxford: Oxford University Press.
3. Moro, M. L., and A. McCormick. Surveillance for communicable disease. In: Eylenbosch, W. J., and N. D. Noah. 1988. *Surveillance in Health and Disease*, 166–182. Oxford: Oxford University Press.
4. Hartgerink, M. J. 1976. Health surveillance and planning for health care in the Netherlands. *Int J Epidemiol* 5:87–91.
5. Editorial. 1976. Surveillance. *Int J Epidemiol* 5:3–6.
6. Langmuir, A. D. 1963. The surveillance of communicable diseases of national importance. *NEJM* 268:182–192.
7. Langmuir, A. D. 1976. William Farr: founder of modern concepts of surveillance. *Int J Epidemiol* 5:13–18.
8. Hinman, A. R. 1972. Surveillance of communicable diseases. Paper presented at the 100th annual meeting of the American Public Health Association, November 15, Atlantic City, New Jersey.
9. National Office of Vital Statistics. 1959. *Vital Statistics of the United States, 1958*. Washington, D.C.
10. Trask, J. W. 1915. Vital statistics: a discussion of what they are and their uses in public health administration. *Public Health Rep* Suppl 12.
11. Bowditch, H. I., D. L. Webster, J. C. Hoadley et al. 1915. Letter from the Massachusetts State Board of Health to physicians. *Public Health Rep* Suppl 12:31.
12. Centers for Disease Control. 1985. *Manual of Procedures for National Morbidity Reporting and Public Health Surveillance Activities*. Atlanta, Ga.: CDC.
13. Chapin, C. V. 1916. State health organization. *JAMA* 66:699–703.
14. National Office of Vital Statistics. 1953. *Reported Incidence of Selected Notifiable Diseases: United States, Each Division and State, 1920–50, Vital Statistics Special Reports—National Summaries*. 37:1180–1181.
15. Langmuir, A. D., N. Nathanson, and W. J. Hall. 1956. Surveillance of poliomyelitis in the United States in 1955. *Am J Public Health* 46:75–88.
16. Nathanson, N., and A. D. Langmuir. 1963. The Cutter incident: poliomyelitis following formaldehyde-inactivated polio virus vaccination in the United States during the spring of 1955. I. Background. *Am J Hyg* 78:29–81.
17. Chorba, T. L., R. L. Berkelman, S. K. Safford, N. P. Gibbs, and H. F. Hull.

1989. The reportable diseases. I. Mandatory reporting of infectious diseases by clinicians. *JAMA* 262: 3018–3026.

18. Langmuir, A. D. 1971. Evolution of the concept of surveillance in the United States. *Proc R Soc Med* 64:681–689.

19. Henderson, D. A. 1980. Smallpox eradication. Public Health Rep 95:422–46.

20. World Health Organization. May 1968. *Report of the Technical Discussions at the Twenty-first World Health Assembly on "National and Global Surveillance of Communicable Diseases,"* A21/Technical Discussions/5. Geneva: WHO.

21. *Int J Epidemiol* (entire issue). 1976. 5:3–91.

22. Raska, K. 1966. National and international surveillance of communicable diseases. *WHO Chron* 20:315–21.

23. World Health Organization. 1963. *Report for Drafting Committee: Terminology of Malaria and of Malaria Eradication.* Geneva: WHO.

24. Retailliau, H. F., A. C. Curtis, G. Starr et al. 1980. Illness after influenza vaccination reported through a nationwide surveillance system, 1976–1977. *Am J Epidemiol* 111:270–278.

25. Schonberger, L. B., D. J. Bregman, J. Z. Sullivan-Bolyai et al. 1979. Guillain-Barré syndrome following vaccination in the National Influenza Immunization Program, United States, 1976–1977. *Am J Epidemiol* 110;105–123.

26. Centers for Disease Control. 1980. *Guillain-Barré Syndrome Surveillance Report, January 1978–March 1979.* Atlanta, Ga.: CDC.

27. Erickson, J. D., J. Mulinare, P. W. McClain et al. 1984. Vietnam veterans' risks for fathering babies with birth defects. *JAMA* 252:903–912.

28. Shands, K. N., G. P. Schmid, B. B. Dan et al. 1980. Toxic shock syndrome in menstruating women. *NEJM* 303:1436–1442.

29. Waldman, R. J., W. N. Hall, H. McGee et al. 1982. Aspirin as a risk factor in Reye syndrome. *JAMA* 247:3089–3094.

30. Centers for Disease Control. 1983. Cancer and steroid hormone study: long-term oral contraceptive use and the risk of breast cancer. *JAMA* 249:1591–1595.

31. Jaffe, H. W., K. Choi, P. A. Thomas et al. 1983. National case-control study of Kaposi's sarcoma and *Pneumocystis carinii* pneumonia in homosexual men: epidemiologic results. *Ann Intern Med* 99:293–298.

32. Thacker, S. B., and R. L. Berkelman. 1988. Public health surveillance in the United States. *Epidemiol Rev* 10:164–190.

33. Berkelman, R. L., and J. W. Buehler. 1988. Public health surveillance of non-infectious chronic diseases: the potential for rapid change in disease burden. Int J Epidemiol 1990; 19:628–34.

34. Baker, E. L., J. M. Melius, and J. D. Millar. 1988. Surveillance of occupational illness and injury in the United States: current perspectives and future directions. *J Public Health Pol* 9:198–221.

35. Muldoon, J. T., L. A. Wintermeyer, J. A. Eure et al. 1987. Occupational disease surveillance data sources, 1985. *Am J Public Health* 77:1006–1008.

36. Centers for Disease Control. 1982. Annual summary 1981: reported morbidity and mortality in the United States. *MMWR* 30:112–113.

37. Edmonds, L. D., P. M. Layde, L. M. James et al. 1981. Congenital malformations surveillance: two American systems. *Int J Epidemiol* 10:247–252.
38. Graitcer, P. L. 1988. The development of state and local injury surveillance systems. *J Safety Res* 18:191–198.
39. Guyer, B., S. S. Gallagher, and C. V. Azzara. 1985. Injury surveillance: a state perspective. *Public Health Rep* 100:588–591.
40. Centers for Disease Control. 1988. Acute traumatic spinal cord injury surveillance: United States, 1987. *MMWR* 37:285–286.
41. Ing, R. T. 1985. Surveillance in injury prevention. *Public Health Rep* 100:586–588.
42. National Center for Health Statistics. 1986. *Health Promotion Data for the 1990 Objectives: Estimates from the National Health Interview Survey of Health Promotion and Disease Prevention, United States, 1985.* Hyattsville, Md.: NCHS. (Advance data from vital and health statistics. Series no. 126; DHHS publication no. (PHS) 86-1250.)
43. Marks, J. S., G. C. Hogelin, E. M. Gentry et al. 1985. The behavioral risk factor surveys. I. State-specific prevalence estimates of behavioral risk factors. *Am J Prev Med* 1:1–8.
44. Thacker, S. B., and R. L. Berkelman. 1986. Surveillance of medical technologies. *J Public Health Pol* 7:363–377.
45. Faich, G. A., D. Knapp, M. Dreis et al. 1987. National adverse drug reaction surveillance: 1985. *JAMA* 257:2068–2070.
46. Royal College of General Practitioners. 1977. Collective research in general practice: influenza. *J R Coll Gen Pract* 27:544–551.
47. Stroobant, A., J. M. Lamotte, V. Van Casteren et al. 1986. Epidemiological surveillance measles through a network of sentinel general practitioners in Belgium. *Int J Epidemiol* 15:386–391.
48. Valleron, A. J., E. Bouvet, P. Garnerin et al. 1986. A computer network for the surveillance of communicable diseases: the French experiment. *Am J Public Health* 76:1289–1292.
49. Graitcer, P. L., and S. B. Thacker. 1986. The French connection. *Am J Public Health* 76:1285–1286.
50. Choi, K., and S. B. Thacker. 1981. An evaluation of influenza mortality surveillance, 1962–1979. I. Time series forecasts of expected pneumonia and influenza deaths. *Am J Epidemiol* 113:215–226.
51. Newhouse, V. F., K. Choi, L. J. D'Angelo et al. 1986. Analysis of social and environmental factors affecting the occurrence of Rocky Mountain spotted fever in Georgia, 1961–1975. *Public Health Rep* 101:419–428.
52. Longini, I. M., Jr., P. E. M. Fine, and S. B. Thacker. 1986. Predicting the global spread of new infectious agents. *Am J Epidemiol* 123:383–391.
53. Thacker, S. B., R. L. Berkelman, and D. F. Stroup. 1989. The science of public health surveillance. *J Public Health Pol* 10:187–203.
54. Thacker, S. B., R. G. Parrish, and F. L. Trowbridge. 1988. A method to evaluate systems of epidemiologic surveillance. *World Health Stat Q* 41:11–18.

2

Surveillance: The Sentinel Health Event Approach

Paul J. Seligman and Todd M. Frazier

A *sentinel health event* is a case of unnecessary disease, unnecessary disability, or untimely death whose occurrence is a warning signal that the quality of preventive or medical care may need to be improved.[1] The purpose of this chapter is to describe the role of sentinel health events in the history of disease and hazard surveillance. In doing this we will describe the development of the concept of sentinel health events—and its precursor, end results analyses—over the past 70 years. We will then illustrate current use in the surveillance of occupational disease and workplace hazards.

Two related but different approaches used in surveillance came from Langmuir and Rutstein. Thacker has described Langmuir's pioneering work; here we will focus on its relationship to the approach taken by his friend and colleague Rutstein. In brief, the contribution to surveillance from Langmuir (by way of Farr) consists of

> the collection of relevant facts, assembling and evaluating them and reporting them to the general public and to responsible health authorities. In Farr's view "the responsibility for enforcing control measures 'belonged to' the official health authority."*

Rutstein's approach starts with the concept of improving the quality of medical care using as a measurement of quality indices based on the counts of cases of unnecessary death, disability, or disease. In 1976, he presented a list of sentinel health events, the occurrence of which noted a failure in

---

* Langmuir, A.D. William Farr: Founder of Modern Concepts of Surveillance: International Journal of Epidemiology Vol. 5: No. 1 1976

the medical delivery system.[1] He acknowledged that the system was not new; it had been used in the "classic studies of maternal mortality of the New York Academy of Medicine in the early 1930's." An earlier application of a similar concept can be attributed to Ernest Amory Codman.

MEDICAL RECORDS

In 1913 Codman proposed an *end result system* "so simple as to seem childlike."[2] The system as proposed by Codman sought answers to this series of questions for each patient seen on the surgical service of a hospital:

What was the matter?
Did they find out beforehand?
Did the patient get entirely well?
If not—why not?
Was it the fault of the surgeon, the disease, or the patient?
What can we do to prevent similar failures in the future?

Codman believed that the practice of medicine and surgery "will always be to a certain extent experimental. . . . The public is entitled to know the results of the experiments it must endure." Instead of answers, Codman's system evoked a reaction from the Boston medical community that resulted in his resignation from the faculty at the Harvard Medical School and from the staff of the Massachusetts General Hospital.[3] Nevertheless, Codman left a significant mark. His work led to the formation of the Joint Commission of Accreditation of Hospitals. Moreover, according to Moore, "Today's concepts of the problem-oriented record, peer review panels, Professional Service Review Organizations . . . and the whole concept of upgrading the quality of medical and surgical care by having doctors examine each other's work in a realistic and objective way traces back to Codman."[3]

VITAL RECORDS

The investigation of surgical deaths pointed the way toward studies of other unfortunate episodes, some of which can appropriately be labeled as "therapeutic misadventures." Examples include the New York Academy of Medicine maternal mortality studies; the pioneering work of Bundesen, Health Commissioner of Chicago, in his studies of natal day deaths; and the anesthetic mortality studies of Phillips in Baltimore.[4]

The link between clinical practice and public health is apparent in this work. Phillips was the chief of the anesthesia department at the Hospital for the Women of Maryland in 1953 when the Medical Society and the Health Department created the Baltimore Anesthesia Study Committee. The charge to the committee, chaired by Phillips, was to "undertake a study of the causes of deaths and other sequelae during and following surgical and obstetrical procedures in the City of Baltimore with a view toward ascertaining the primary causes of these mishaps. . . ."[5]

Death certificates of all persons whose deaths occurred the day of or the day after an operative procedure initiated a case study based on the hospital's medical records and, in some cases, a medical examiner's report. These were the sentinel health events. The collection of and discussion by Study Committee members of information on 1,024 postoperative deaths in Baltimore, and the analysis of the clinical and medical examiner's review of these sentinel health events, resulted in the finding that anesthetic management contributed to nearly 20 percent of these deaths. This, along with the observation that half of these deaths occurred in patients' rooms following the operation, presented "a strong case for the routine utilization of postanesthetic areas where facilities for intensive observation and care" would be constantly available.[4] The dissemination of this information to the medical community, the public health authority, and hospital boards contributed to the development of the postoperative recovery rooms that we have today.

SENTINEL EVENTS: CURRENT USE

The use of public health systems of vital events and reportable disease in conjunction with medical records and case reports formed what Rutstein called *quality control systems*.[6]

> Two different kinds of control systems will be needed to collect, analyze, and feed back those data on the quality of care that are essential to the administration of an effective national health program . . . ; a guidance system to measure, follow and interpret accomplishments and failures, and to lay out a course for future programs; and an early warning system to identify sudden outcroppings of undesirable health events that may demand immediate action. Both systems will focus on the occurrence of unnecessary disease, disability, and untimely death as negative indices of the quality of medical care. The guidance system will determine and compare their statistical distribution throughout the country and in each medical care region, while the early warning system will signal and evaluate the epidemiological occurrence of the individual sentinel events.

The two approaches—the guidance system akin to the Langmuir-Farr approach and Rutstein's early warning system—form a surveillance model that conforms to the Center for Disease Control's (CDC) definition for public health surveillance. It utilizes ongoing systems for the collection, analysis, and interpretation of health data, and is used in the planning, implementation, and evaluation of clinical and public health practice.

The two-part approach appears to be most effective when clinical and public health practitioners understand their symbiotic roles. The examples of the joint efforts of clinical and public health practice in the development of surveillance systems set the stage for the implementation of intervention strategies, such as prenatal care, neonatology, and postoperative recovery rooms.

Rutstein's sentinel health event (SHE) concept has now been adapted to meet the needs for surveillance in occupational health. In 1978 one of us (TMF) met with Dr. David Rutstein, who at that time was the Ridley Watts Professor of Preventive Medicine Emeritus, to discuss the idea of applying his sentinel health event concept to the field of occupational health. He was enthusiastic about this and for the next several years served as a consultant to the National Institute for Occupational Safety and Health (NIOSH) in a project that resulted in the publication of a list of 50 disease rubrics that are called Sentinel Health Events (Occupational).[7]

In this list we included "only those conditions . . . for which objective documentation of an associated agent, industry, and occupation existed in the scientific literature." The list was developed to serve as a basis for physician recognition and public health surveillance. Based on the previous experience with maternal and infant mortality, we were convinced that, with appropriate modification, the SHE concept could be successfully applied to the field of occupational disease. Thus we have defined the Sentinel Health Event (Occupational), or SHE(O), as: an unnecessary "disease, disability, or untimely death which is occupationally related and whose occurrence may (1) provide the impetus for epidemiologic or industrial hygiene studies; or (2) serve as a warning signal that materials substitution, engineering control, personal protection, or medical care may be required." This list of Sentinel Health Events has recently been updated.[8]

The components for successful application of the Sentinel Health Event approach appear to include

1. an identifiable end result or sentinel event
2. a surveillance system for collection of relevant data and its analysis and dissemination
3. the cooperation of medical care providers and public health authorities
4. the successful implementation of an effective intervention strategy

APPLICATION OF THE SENTINEL HEALTH EVENT APPROACH: UNNECESSARY DISEASE, UNNECESSARY DISABILITY, UNTIMELY DEATH

In the realm of environmental and occupational diseases, are any manmade diseases really "necessary" in the sense that they are unavoidable? With the application of technology to control exposures, all health conditions secondary to exposures to chemical, physical, or biological agents generated in the manufacturing or processing of goods and materials are potentially avoidable. Citing the success of the smallpox eradication effort, Rutstein notes that where "scientific evidence of preventability is clear, it is possible to surmount bureaucratic inertia, deeply rooted prejudices, careless indifference, and economic barriers and obtain widespread cooperation to implement a centrally directed, locally operated, carefully devised plan to eradicate, control, or reduce the impact of a preventable disease."[9]

OCCUPATIONAL DISEASE SURVEILLANCE: "70 YEARS BEHIND"

Testifying before a subcommittee of the House Committee on Government Operations in 1984, J. Donald Millar, director of NIOSH, stated that "in the practice of epidemiologic surveillance, the field of occupational safety and health is at least 70 years behind the field of communicable disease control."[10] Dr. Millar's observation was based on the fact that in 1912 the Conference of State and Territorial Health Authorities recommended "weekly telegraphic reporting to the Federal Government of selected communicable diseases." These routine reports have become a vital component in disease monitoring and control nationwide with the summary of these reports appearing in the *Morbidity and Mortality Weekly Report* (*MMWR*). In 1986, noting that the United States is the "only large developed country without a national system for reporting occupational disease" and that the Conference of State and Territorial Epidemiologists supported national reporting of selected occupational diseases, the same Congressional subcommittee recommended that the CDC "require reporting of occupational illnesses in all 50 states."[11]

SENTINEL HEALTH EVENT APPROACH: CURRENT CONCEPTS IN OCCUPATIONAL DISEASE SURVEILLANCE

The developmental points of the sentinel health event approach—the components of surveillance from Farr and Langmuir to Codman and Rutstein—are exemplified by current efforts to build surveillance systems for occupational injuries and illnesses. Lead poisoning surveillance in the workplace exemplifies the synthesis of many of these principles, and highlights the main features in successful attempts at applying public health models developed in the areas of infectious disease to occupational health.

The similarities between the sentinel approach to a public health problem in a clinical setting and the assessment of a workplace hazard and its health effects provide important guidance and the foundation for future efforts in building successful occupational disease surveillance programs. The Sentinel Event Notification Systems for Occupational Risk (SENSOR) program at NIOSH is based on principles articulated by Codman and Rutstein.[12] These principles include

1. a case-based approach to surveillance
2. the immediate application of surveillance information to prevention activities

Intervention activities start with field investigations to identify the source of the disease. Onsite evaluation offers the opportunity to identify additional cases, determine the degree of the hazardous exposure, and provide technical guidance to correct the problem at that worksite. Information gathered in the course of field investigations may be used to identify problems particular to a process that occurs throughout industry. Investigation of one case at one plant may have impact for an entire industry. For example, cases of lead poisoning among radiator repair workers led to the recognition of lead exposure as a nationwide problem, and resulted in the formulation and application of control technologies to control lead exposures in that industry.[13, 14]

Follow-up of a sentinel health event allows for immediate feedback to the clinician and provides a direct link between the clinical and public health communities. In 1984, a cooperative effort between NIOSH and The Industrial Commission of Ohio examined the utility of workers' compensation claims for the surveillance of occupational lead poisoning.[15] While the numbers of compensation claims for this condition are few compared to the numbers of workers overexposed to lead at the workplace, the practical lessons learned during the analysis and follow-up of these claims serve as examples of the applicability of the sentinel health event approach to the surveillance of this still common problem.[16] It demonstrates how this approach is applied in the description and assessment of a common manmade disease (lead poisoning) in the work environment.

For occupational lead poisoning, the evidence for its preventability is the basis for the 1978 Occupational Safety and Health Administration's Lead Standard, which at that time based its permissible exposure limits on the reduction of exposures to levels below which health effects were observed in adult workers.[17] The average length of disability for lead poisoning claims in the compensation system in Ohio was 60 days, clearly unnecessary in the face of its being preventable by exposure control. While deaths from acute lead poisoning were common in Ohio in the early twentieth century,[18] these events are now exceedingly rare and are usually found in the context of intentional ingestion, inadvertent administration of folk medicines high in lead content, or use of tainted illicit methamphetamine. The magnitude of the contribution of a lifetime of industrial or environmental lead exposure to chronic renal disease, hypertension, and premature cardiovascular morbidity and mortality is currently unknown.

For the five-year period, 1979 to 1983, 114 compensation claims for lead poisoning were filed with the Ohio Bureau of Workers' Compensation. Of these 114 claims, 92 (81 percent) met a case definition for lead poisoning. Thirty companies accounted for these cases: Previous OSHA inspections had occurred at 14 of them. NIOSH conducted site visits at seven of the remaining 16 worksites to determine whether ongoing lead hazards existed, what the company was doing to remedy the hazards, and whether there were cases of elevated blood lead levels among the workforce that were not reported to the workers' compensation system. Applying Codman's criteria we asked the following questions:

What Was the Matter?

Five of the companies evaluated were not aware of the degree of the lead hazard at the time of the compensation claim. One company was not aware that lead was in one of the products they were using and one company was aware of the lead problem, but was having difficulty controlling it.

Did They Find Out Beforehand?

Six of the seven companies were not aware that they had a lead exposure problem prior to the compensation claims. In all companies evaluated, additional cases of lead poisoning were identified.

Did the Patient Get Well?

The compensation claims resulted in a decrease in the blood lead levels in five of the worksites. In one worksite, no reduction was observed, and in one plant, the workers who had filed compensation claims were not available for follow-up. In five of the plants, exposure conditions had improved; in two they had not. Where exposure conditions had not improved, one plant appeared to lack the financial resources to fix the problem; the other a lack of will to improve working conditions.

Whose Fault Was It?

In examining the issue of "fault" in occupational health, one must examine the attributes of the disease, the work environment provided by the management of the company, and the work practices of the individuals performing the job. For a manmade disease like lead poisoning, where the degree of contact with the material is controlled by the characteristics of the process, little fault can be placed on the "disease" per se. The one possible exception to this is where technologies do not exist or are unavailable to control exposures. In occupational health, limiting hazardous exposures through engineering controls, use of personal protective equipment, and provision of and adherence to an industrial hygiene program are management mainstays in the creation of a healthy and safe work environment. The potential contribution of a worker's personal habits (e.g., smoking) and hygiene must also be considered in evaluating the source of an occupational disease.

What Can We Do to Prevent Similar Failures in the Future?

In occupational health, multiple tiers exist to prevent cases of occupational disease from occurring in the future. The layers of intervention/prevention include (1) the education of both the worker and management, (2) the provision of a health care structure to monitor the health and safety of the work environment, (3) the participation of public health authorities charged with the responsibility of investigating cases of occupational diseases, and (4) an intervention strategy that recommends changes to render the work environment hazard-free.

CONCLUSION

In occupational health, the surveillance of hazardous agents, or "hazard surveillance," has a unique and important role in identifying worksites where potential health hazards may exist.[19] The knowledge of hazards and their control form the first step in the prevention of occupational diseases.[20] Because of their pervasiveness in the work environment (e.g., inorganic lead), or because of the health risks that they pose years after cessation from exposure (e.g., asbestos), a number of agents merit hazard surveillance, which would form the basis for a case report in a "sentinel" event surveillance system in the absence of overt disease. An area for future efforts in the area of occupational health is the development of a list of "sentinel hazards" similar to the existing list of "sentinel health events."

The sentinel event approach is distinctly different from surveillance that monitors trends in disease based on population-based rates. The end result or sentinel event approach (Codman and Rutstein) is distinct from the surveillance that monitors trends in disease based on population-based rates (Farr and Langmuir). In surveillance two related approaches were used: one population-based, the other case-based. The accumulation of cases (end results or sentinel events) can, in some circumstances, provide a database for monitoring trends. Thus, the distinction between the Farr–Langmuir and Codman–Rutstein approaches as described here is blurred. Together they provide methods that are basic in public health. The success of public health activities depends on its ability to not only demonstrate an impact on the reduction of disease and disability, but also "fight the fires" as they erupt. The sentinel health event approach is simply the firefighting mechanism that complements rate-based trend surveillance.

Notes

1. Rutstein, D. D., W. Berenberg, T. C. Chalmers, C. G. Child, A. P. Fishman, and E. B. Perrin. 1976. Measuring the quality of medical care: a clinical method. *NEJM* 294:582–588.
2. Codman, E. A. 1916. *A Study in Hospital Efficiency.* Boston: Thomas Todd Co.
3. Moore, F. D. 1975. Surgical biology and applied sociology: Cannon and Codman fifty years later. *Harvard Medical Alumni Bull* 49(3):12–21.
4. Phillips, O. C., T. M. Frazier, T. D. Graff, T. J. DeKornfeld. 1960. The Baltimore Anesthesia Study Committee: a review of 1,024 postoperative deaths. *JAMA* 174:2015–2019.
5. Phillips, O. C., and T. M. Frazier. 1957. The Baltimore Anesthesia Study Committee organization and preliminary report. *Anesthesiology* 18:33–43.
6. Rutstein, D. D. 1974. *Blueprint for Medical Care.* Cambridge, Massachusetts and London, England: The MIT Press. 174.
7. Rutstein, D. D., R. J. Mullan, T. M. Frazier, W. E. Halperin, J. M. Melius, and J. P. Sestito. 1983. Sentinel health events (occupational): a basis for physician recognition and public health surveillance. *Am J Public Health* 73:1054–1062.
8. Mullan, R. J., and L. I. Murthy. 1991. Occupational sentinel health events: an updated list for physician recognition and public health surveillance. *Am J Ind Med* 19:775–799.

9. Rutstein, D. D. 1981. Controlling the communicable and man-made diseases. *NEJM* 304:1422–1424.
10. Millar, D. J. 1984. OSHA Injury and Illness Information System. Testimony before a Subcommittee of the Committee on Government Operations, House of Representatives, June 20, 98th Cong. 2d sess.
11. Occupational Health Hazard Surveillance: 72 Years Behind and Counting. 1986. 61st Report by Committee on Governmental Operations, Together with Additional and Supplemental Views. 99th Cong. 2nd Session House Report 99-979, October 8.
12. Baker, E. L. 1989. Sentinel Event Notification System for Occupational Risks (SENSOR): The Concept. *Am J Public Health* 79(supp):18–20.
13. Goldman, R. H., E. L. Baker, M. Hannan et al. 1987. Lead poisoning in automobile radiator mechanics. *NEJM* 317:214–218.
14. Centers for Disease Control. 1991. Control of excessive lead exposure in radiator repair workers. *MMWR* 40:139–141.
15. Seligman, P. J., W. E. Halperin, R. J. Mullan, and T. M. Frazier. 1986. Occupational lead poisoning in Ohio: surveillance using workers' compensation data. *Am J Public Health* 76:1299–1302.
16. Seligman, P. J., and W. E. Halperin. 1991. Targeting of workplace inspections for lead. *Am J Ind Med* 20:381–390.
17. U.S. Department of Labor, Occupational Safety and Health Administration. Standard for Occupational Exposure to Lead (29 CFR 1910.1025). 1985.
18. Hayhurst, E. R. 1915. *A Survey of Industrial Health-Hazards and Occupational Diseases in Ohio*. Ohio State Board of Health. Columbus, Ohio. The F.J. Heer Printing Co.
19. Sundin, D. S., D. H. Pedersen, and T. M. Frazier. 1986. Occupational hazard and health surveillance. *Am J Public Health* 76:1083–1084.
20. Halperin, W. E., and T. M. Frazier. 1985. Surveillance for the effects of workplace exposure. *Ann Rev Public Health* 6:419–432.

3

Evaluating Public Health Surveillance Systems

Douglas N. Klaucke

Public health surveillance is the ongoing and systematic collection, analysis, and interpretation of health data to describe and monitor a health event. This information is then used for planning, implementing, and evaluating public health interventions and programs. Surveillance data are used both to determine the need for public health action and to assess the effectiveness of programs.

The purpose of evaluating surveillance systems is to promote the best use of public health resources by ensuring that only important problems are under surveillance and that surveillance systems operate efficiently. The evaluation of surveillance systems, to the extent possible, should recommend improvements in quality and efficiency, such as by eliminating unnecessary duplication. Most important, an evaluation should assess whether a system is serving a useful public health function and is meeting the system's objectives.

Because surveillance systems vary widely in their methods, scope, and objectives, characteristics that are important to one system may be less important to another. Efforts to improve certain attributes—such as the ability of a system to detect a health event—may detract from other attributes, such as simplicity or timeliness. Thus, the success of an individual surveillance system depends on the proper balance of characteristics, and the strength of an evaluation depends on the ability of the evaluator to assess these characteristics with respect to the system's objectives. In an effort to accommodate these objectives, any approach to evaluation must be flexible. With this in mind, the methods discussed in this chapter must be applied discriminately; all measures will not be appropriate for all systems.

26

PUBLIC HEALTH IMPORTANCE

The first step in evaluating a surveillance system is to describe the public health importance of the event(s) under surveillance. The public health importance of a health event and the need to have that health event under surveillance can be described in a variety of ways. Health events that affect many people or require large expenditures of resources clearly have public health importance. However, health events that affect relatively few persons may also be important, especially if the events cluster in time and place, such as in a limited outbreak of a severe disease. At other times, public concerns may focus attention on a particular health event, creating or heightening its sense of importance. Diseases that are now rare due to successful control measures may be perceived as "unimportant," but their level of importance should be assessed in light of their potential to reemerge. Finally, the public health importance of the health event is influenced by its preventability. Parameters for measuring the importance of a health event and, therefore, the surveillance system that monitors it include:

1. The total number of cases, indicating incidence and prevalence
2. Indices of severity, such as the mortality rate and the case-fatality ratio
3. An index of lost productivity, such as bed disability days
4. An index of premature mortality, such as years of potential life lost (YPLL)
5. Medical costs
6. Preventability

These measures of importance do not take into account the effect of existing control measures. For example, although the number of cases of vaccine-preventable illness has declined following the implementation of school immunization laws, the public health importance of these diseases would be underestimated by case counts alone. In such instances, it may be possible to estimate the number of cases that would be expected in the absence of control programs.[1]

Preventability can be defined at several levels: preventing the occurrence of disease (primary prevention); employing early detection and intervention with the aim of reversing, halting, or at least retarding the progress of a condition (secondary prevention); and minimizing the effects of disease and disability among the already ill (tertiary prevention). From the perspective of surveillance, preventability reflects the potential for effective public health interventions at any of these levels.

Attempts have been made to quantify the public health importance of various diseases and health conditions. Dean et al. described such an approach using a score that took into account age-specific mortality and morbidity rates and health care costs.[2]

SYSTEM DESCRIPTION

The next step is to describe the system. The following four tasks are involved:

1. List the objectives of the system.
2. Describe the health event(s) under surveillance. State the case definition for each of the health events.
3. Describe the components and operation of the system.
4. Draw a flow chart of the system.

Objectives may include detecting or monitoring outbreaks, monitoring trends, identification of contacts and administration of prophylaxis, enrolling cases in a study, generating hypotheses about etiology, and so forth. The objectives of the system define a framework for evaluating the specific components.

Next, describe the components of a surveillance system. This can be done by answering the following questions:

1. What is the population under surveillance?
2. What is the period of time of the data collection?
3. What information is collected?
4. Who provides the surveillance information?
5. How is the information transferred?
6. How is the information stored?
7. Who analyzes the data?
8. How are the data analyzed, and how often?
9. Are there preliminary and final tabulations, analyses, and reports?
10. How often are reports disseminated?
11. To whom are reports distributed?
12. How are the reports distributed?

It is often useful to list the discrete steps in the processing of health event reports by the system, and then to depict these steps in a flow chart (see Fig. 3-1).

USEFULNESS

The third step is to describe the usefulness of the system.

1. Describe the actions that have been taken as a result of the data from the surveillance system.
2. Describe the personnel who have used the data to make decisions and take actions.
3. List other anticipated uses of the data.

A surveillance system is useful if it contributes to the control and prevention of adverse health events, including an improved understanding of the public health implications of such events. A surveillance system can also be useful if it determines that an adverse health event initially thought to be important is not.

An assessment of the usefulness of a surveillance system begins with a review of the objectives of the system and should consider the dependence of policy decisions and control measures on surveillance. Depending on the objectives of a particular surveillance system, the system may be considered useful if it satisfactorily addresses one or more of the following questions. Does the system:

1. Detect trends signaling changes in the occurrence of disease?
2. Detect epidemics?
3. Provide estimates of the magnitude of morbidity and mortality related to the health problem under surveillance?
4. Stimulate epidemiologic research likely to lead to control or prevention?
5. Identify risk factors involved in disease occurrence?
6. Permit assessment of the effects of control measures?
7. Lead to improved clinical practice by the health care providers who are the constituents of the surveillance system?

Usefulness may be affected by all the attributes of surveillance. Increased sensitivity may afford a greater opportunity for identifying epidemics and understanding the natural course of an adverse health event in a community. Improved timeliness allows earlier control and prevention activities. Increased specificity enables the public health officials to focus on productive activities. A representative surveillance system will better characterize the

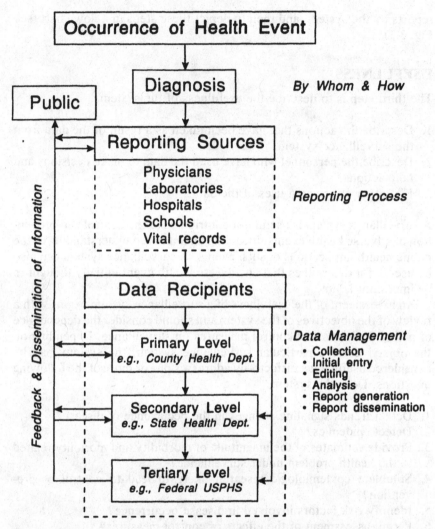

FIGURE 3-1.   The major steps in a public health surveillance system.

epidemiologic characteristics of a health event in the population. Systems that are simple, flexible, and acceptable will also tend to be more useful.

SYSTEM ATTRIBUTES

The fourth step is to evaluate the system for each of the following attributes:

1. Simplicity
2. Flexibility
3. Acceptability
4. Sensitivity
5. Predictive Value Positive
6. Representativeness
7. Timeliness

Simplicity

The simplicity of a surveillance system refers to both its structure and its ease of operation. While surveillance systems should be as simple as possible, they must still meet their objectives.

A chart describing the flow of information and the lines of response in a surveillance system can help assess the simplicity or complexity of a surveillance system. A flow chart for a generic surveillance system is illustrated in Figure 3-1. The following measures might be considered in evaluating the simplicity of a system:

1. Amount and type of information necessary to establish the diagnosis
2. Number and type of reporting sources
3. Method(s) of transmitting case information/data
4. Number of organizations involved in receiving case reports
5. Staff training requirements
6. Type and extent of data analysis
7. Number and type of users of compiled case information
8. Method of distributing reports or case information to these users
9. Time spent on the following tasks:

   a. Maintaining the system
   b. Collecting case information
   c. Transmitting case information
   d. Analyzing case information
   e. Preparing and disseminating surveillance reports

It may be useful to consider the simplicity of a surveillance system from two major perspectives: the design of the system and the size of the system. An example of a system that is simple in design is one where the case definition is easy to apply and where the person identifying the case will also be the one analyzing and using the information. A more complex system might involve the following:

- Special laboratory tests required to confirm the case.
- Telephone contact or a home visit by a public health nurse to collect detailed information.
- Multiple levels of reporting. For example, with the notifiable diseases reporting system, case reports may start with the doctor who makes the diagnosis, and pass through county and state health departments before referral to the Centers for Disease Control.

Simplicity is closely related to the attribute of timeliness, and will affect the amount of resources that are required to operate the system.

Flexibility

A flexible surveillance system can adapt to changing information needs or operating conditions with little additional cost in time, personnel, or funds. Flexible systems can accommodate, for example, new diseases and health conditions, changes in case definitions, changes in the amount and type of information collected, and variations in reporting sources.

Flexibility is probably best judged in hindsight, by observing how a system responded to a new demand. For example, when AIDS emerged in 1981, the existing notifiable disease reporting system of state health departments was used to report cases. AIDS surveillance has since been adapted to rapidly advancing knowledge about the disease, its diagnosis, and its risk factors. Another example is the capacity of the gonorrhea surveillance system to accommodate special surveillance for penicillinase-producing Neisseria gonorrhoeae. Unless efforts have been made to adapt a system to another disease, it may be difficult to assess the flexibility of a system. In the absence of practical experience, one can look at the design and workings of a system.

Acceptability

Acceptability reflects the willingness of individuals and organizations to participate in the surveillance system. This attribute refers to the acceptability of the system to persons outside the sponsoring agency, such as those who are being asked to do something for the system, and to persons within the sponsoring agency who are operating the system. To assess acceptability, one must consider the points of interaction between the system and its participants, including subjects (persons identified as cases) and those reporting cases. Quantitative indicators of acceptability include:

- Subject or agency participation rates

TABLE 3-1

		"Condition" Present		
		YES	NO	
	YES	True Positive A	False Positive B	A + B
Detected by Surveillance				
	NO	False Negative C	True Negative D	C + D
		A + C	B + D	Total

Sensitivity = A/(A + C)
Predictive Value Positive = A/(A + B)

- Interview completion rates and question refusal rates, if the system involves case interviews
- Completeness of report forms
- Physician, laboratory, or hospital/facility reporting rates
- Timeliness of reporting

Some of these measures may be obtained from a review of surveillance report forms, while others would require special studies or surveys.

Acceptability is a largely subjective attribute that encompasses the willingness of persons on whom the system depends to provide accurate, consistent, complete, and timely data. Some factors influencing the acceptability of a particular system are:

- The public health importance of the health event
- Recognition by the system of the individual's contribution
- Responsiveness of the system to suggestions or comments
- Time burden relative to available time
- Federal and state legislative restrictions on data collection and ensurance of confidentiality
- Federal and state legislative requirements for reporting

Sensitivity

The sensitivity of a surveillance system can be considered on two levels. First, at the level of case reporting, the proportion of cases of a disease or health condition that are detected by the surveillance system (Table 3-1) can be evaluated. Second, the system can be evaluated for its ability to detect epidemics.[3]

The sensitivity of a surveillance system is affected by the likelihood that

1. persons with certain diseases or health conditions seek medical care;
2. the diseases or conditions will be correctly diagnosed, reflecting the skill of care providers and the accuracy of diagnostic tests;
3. the case will be reported to the system, given the diagnosis.

These questions can be extended by analogy to surveillance systems that do not fit the traditional disease/care provider model. For example, the sensitivity of a telephone-based surveillance system of morbidity or risk factors would be affected by

1. the number of people who have telephones, who are at home when the surveyor calls, and who agree to participate;
2. the ability of persons to understand the questions and correctly identify their status;
3. the willingness of respondents to report their status.

The extent to which these questions are explored depends on the system and on the resources available for the evaluation. The measurement of sensitivity in a surveillance system requires (a) the validation of information collected by the system to distinguish accurate from inaccurate case reports and (b) the collection of information external to the system to determine the frequency of the condition in a community.[1] From a practical standpoint, the primary emphasis in assessing sensitivity, assuming most reported cases are correctly classified, is to estimate what proportion of the total number of cases in the community are being detected by the system.

A surveillance system that does not have high sensitivity can still be useful in monitoring trends, as long as the sensitivity remains reasonably constant. Questions concerning sensitivity in surveillance systems most commonly arise when changes in disease occurrence are noted. Changes in sensitivity can be precipitated by such variables as the heightened awareness of a disease, the introduction of new diagnostic tests, and changes in the method of conducting surveillance. A search for such surveillance "artifacts" is often an initial step in outbreak investigations.

Predictive Value Positive

Predictive value positive (PVP) is the proportion of persons identified as cases who truly have the condition under surveillance.[3] In Table 3-1 this is represented by A/(A + B).

In assessing PVP, primary emphasis is placed on the confirmation of cases reported through the surveillance system. Its effect on the use of public health resources can be considered on two levels. At the level of an individual case PVP affects the amount of resources used for case investigations. For example, in some states every reported case of hepatitis A is promptly investigated by a public health nurse, and family members at risk are referred for a prophylactic immune globulin injection. A surveillance system with low PVP, and therefore frequent "false positive" case reports, would result in wasted resources. The other level is that of epidemic detection. A high rate of erroneous case reports may trigger an inappropriate outbreak investigation. In assessing this attribute we want to know what proportion of epidemics identified by the surveillance system are "true" epidemics."

Calculating the PVP may require that records of all interventions initiated due to information obtained from the surveillance system be kept. A record of the number of case investigations done and the proportion of those that actually had the condition under surveillance would allow the calculation of the PVP at the level of case detection. Personnel activity reports, travel records, and telephone logbooks may all be useful in estimating the PVP at the epidemic detection level.

This rate is important because a low PVP means that (a) noncases are being investigated, and (b) epidemics may be mistakenly identified. "False positive" reports to surveillance systems lead to unnecessary interventions, and falsely detected "epidemics" lead to costly investigations. A surveillance system with high PVP will lead to fewer "wild goose chases" and wasted resources. An example of a surveillance evaluation that examined PVP was done by Barker et al. They reviewed hospital charts to determine the proportion of persons admitted with a diagnosis of stroke who had the diagnosis confirmed.[5] The PVP for a health event is closely related to the clarity and specificity of the case definition. Good communication between the persons who report cases and the receiving agency also can improve PVP. The PVP reflects the sensitivity and specificity of the case definition and the prevalence of the condition in the population (see Table 3-1). The PVP increases with increasing specificity and prevalence.

Representativeness

A surveillance system that is representative accurately describes (a) the occurrence of a health event over time and (b) its distribution in the population by place and person.

Representativeness is assessed by comparing the characteristics of reported events to all such events which occurred. Although this information is generally unknown, some judgment of the representativeness of surveillance data is possible, based on knowledge of the following:

1. Characteristics of the population; for example, socioeconomic status, and geographic location[6]
2. Natural history of the condition, such as latency period or fatal outcome
3. Prevailing medical practices, including sites performing diagnostic tests and physician referral patterns[7, 8]
4. Multiple sources of data, such as mortality rates for comparison with incidence data and laboratory reports for comparison with physician reports

Representativeness could be more carefully examined through special studies which seek to identify a sample of all cases.

Data quality is an important part of representativeness. Much of the discussion in this book focuses on the identification and classification of cases. However, most surveillance systems collect more than simple case counts. Information commonly collected includes the demographic characteristics of affected persons, details about the health event, and the presence or absence of potential risk factors. The quality, usefulness, and representativeness of this information depends on its completeness and validity.

Data quality is influenced by the clarity of forms, the training and supervision of persons who complete surveillance forms, and the care exercised in data management. A review of these facets of a surveillance system would provide an indirect measure of data quality. Examining the percentage of "unknown" or "blank" responses to items on surveillance forms or questionnaires is straightforward. Assessing the validity of responses would require special studies, such as chart reviews or re-interviews of respondents.

In order to generalize findings from surveillance data to the population at large, the data from a surveillance system should reflect the population characteristics that are important to the goals and objectives of that system. These characteristics generally relate to time, place, and person. An important result of evaluating the representativeness of a surveillance system is the identification of population subgroups which may be systematically excluded from the reporting system. This will enable appropriate modification of data collection and more accurate projections of incidence of the health event in the target population.

For example, an evaluation of viral hepatitis reporting in a county in

Washington suggested that cases of hepatitis B were underreported among homosexual men and that cases of hepatitis nonA-nonB were under-reported among persons exposed to blood transfusions. The importance of these risk factors as contributors to the occurrence of these diseases was apparently underestimated by the selective underreporting of certain hepatitis cases.[9]

Errors and bias can make their way into a surveillance system at any stage. Because surveillance data are used to identify high-risk groups and to target and evaluate interventions, it is important to be aware of the strengths and limitations of the information in the system.

Thus far, the discussion of attributes has been aimed at the information collected for cases, but in many surveillance systems morbidity and mortality rates are calculated. The denominators for these rate calculations are often obtained from a completely separate data system that is maintained by another agency such as the Bureau of the Census or the CDC National Center for Health Statistics. Evaluation of the quality of these data is a science in itself but thought should be given to the comparability of categories (e.g., race, age, residence, etc.) used in the numerator and denominator of rate calculations.

Timeliness

Timeliness reflects the speed or delay between any two or more steps in a surveillance system.

The major steps in a surveillance system are shown in Figure 3-1. The time interval between any two of the steps in this figure can be examined. The intervals usually considered first are the amount of time between the onset of an adverse health event and either the report of the event to the public health agency responsible for instituting control and prevention measures or the identification by that agency of trends, outbreaks, or the effect of control measures. With acute diseases the onset of symptoms is usually used. Sometimes the date of exposure is used. With chronic diseases it may be more useful to look at time from diagnosis rather than try to estimate an onset date.

The timeliness of a surveillance system should be evaluated in terms of availability of information for disease control, either for immediate control efforts or for long-term program planning.

For example, a study of a surveillance system for Shigella infections indicated that the typical case of shigellosis was brought to the attention of health officials 11 days after onset of symptoms—a time sufficient for the occurrence of secondary and tertiary transmission. This suggests that timeliness was insufficient for effective disease control.[10] In contrast, when there is a long latency period between exposure and the appearance of disease, the rapid identification of cases of illness may not be as important as the rapid availability of data to interrupt and prevent exposures that lead to disease. On another time frame, surveillance data are being used by public health agencies to track progress toward the 1990 Objectives for the Nation and to plan for the Year 2000 Objectives.

The need for rapidity of response in a surveillance system depends on the nature of the public health problem under surveillance and the objectives of the system. Recently, computer technology has been integrated into surveillance systems and may promote timeliness[11, 12].

RESOURCES FOR SYSTEM OPERATION

The fifth step is to describe the resources that are used to operate the system. Emphasis should be placed on the resources that are directly required to operate the surveillance system. These are sometimes referred to as "direct costs" and include the personnel and financial resources applied to the collection, processing, analysis, and dissemination of the surveillance data. In estimating these resources consider the following:

- Personnel requirements. A first step is to estimate the time it takes to operate the system. This could be expressed as person-time expended per year of operation. If desired, these could be converted to dollar estimates by multiplying the person-time by appropriate salary and benefit figures.
- Other resources. These may include the cost of travel, training, supplies, equipment, and services such as mail, telephone, and computer time.

The application of these resources at all levels of the public health system, from the local health care provider to municipal, county, state, and federal health agencies, should be considered.

The approach to resources described here includes only those personnel and material resources required for the operation of surveillance and excludes a broader definition of costs that might be considered in a more comprehensive evaluation. The estimation of the costs of a surveillance system can be a complex process, including the estimation of (a) indirect costs, such as follow-up laboratory tests or treatments incurred as a result of surveillance, (b) costs of secondary data sources (e.g., vital statistics or survey data), and (c) costs averted (benefits) by surveillance.

Costs are judged in comparison to benefits, but few evaluations of surveillance systems are likely to include a formal cost/benefit analysis, and such analyses are beyond the scope of this book. Estimating benefits,

TABLE 3-2   Comparison of Health Department Estimated Costs for Active and Passive Surveillance Systems, Vermont, June 1, 1980 to May 31, 1981

Cast Categories	Type of Surveillance System	
	Active[1]	Passive[2]
Paper	$ 114	$ 80
Mailing	185	, 48
Telephone	1,947	175
Personnel		
Secretary	3,000	2,000
Public Health Nurses	14,025	0
Total	**$19,271**	**$2,203**

[1] Weekly calls made from health department to request reports.
[2] Provider initiated reporting.

SOURCE: Vogt et al. *Am J Public Health* 1983; 73:795–797.

such as savings resulting from morbidity prevented through surveillance data, may be possible in some instances, although this approach does not take into account the full spectrum of benefits that may result from surveillance systems. More realistically, costs should be judged with respect to the objectives and usefulness of a surveillance system.

For example, a comparison of two methods of collecting surveillance data was made in Vermont. The "passive" system was already in place and consisted of unsolicited reports of notifiable diseases to the district offices or state health department. The "active" system was implemented in a probability sample of physician practices. Each week a health department employee called these practices to solicit reports of selected notifiable diseases. In comparing the two systems an attempt was made to estimate their costs. The resource estimates directly applied to the surveillance systems are shown in Table 3-2.

CONCLUSIONS AND RECOMMENDATIONS

Finally, you should list your conclusions and recommendations. These should state whether the system is addressing an important public health problem and is meeting its objectives. Recommendations should address the continuation and/or modification of the surveillance system.

The attributes and costs of a surveillance system are interdependent.

Before recommending changes in a system, interactions among the attributes and costs should be considered to ensure that benefits from strengthening one attribute would not affect another in an unacceptable way.

Efforts to increase sensitivity, specificity, timeliness, and representativeness tend to increase the cost of a surveillance system, although savings in efficiency with automation may offset some of these costs.[12]

As sensitivity and specificity approach 100 percent, the surveillance system is more likely to be representative of the populations of interest. As sensitivity increases, specificity may decrease if more false positives are reported. Efforts to increase sensitivity and specificity tend to make a surveillance system more complex, potentially decreasing its acceptability, timeliness, and flexibility. For example, a study comparing health department initiated (active) surveillance to provider-initiated (passive) surveillance did not improve timeliness despite increased sensitivity.[8]

In summary, evaluating surveillance systems is not easy. There is no perfect system; trade-offs must always be made. Each system is unique and therefore requires a balancing of the effort and resources put into each of its components if the system is to achieve its intended goal. This chapter presents guidelines—not absolutes—for the evaluation of surveillance systems. Attributes have been described that can be examined and evaluated to assess a system's ability to achieve the objectives for which it was designed. The goal is to make the evaluation process more explicit and objective.

Notes

1. Hinman, A. R., and J. P. Koplan. 1984. Pertussis and pertussis vaccine: reanalysis of benefits, risks, and costs. *JAMA* 251:3109–3113.
2. Dean, A. G., D. J. West, and W. M. Weir. 1982. Measuring loss of life, health, and income due to disease and injury. *Public Health Rep* 97:38–47.
3. Weinstein, M. C., and H. V. Fineberg. 1980. *Clinical Decision Analysis.* Philadelphia: W. B. Saunders Co., 84–94.
4. Chandra Sekar, C., and W. E. Deming. 1949. On a method of estimating birth and death rates and the extent of registration. *J Am Stat Assoc* 44:101–115.
5. Barker, W. H., K. S. Feldt, J. Feibel et al. 1984. Assessment of hospital admission surveillance of stroke in a metropolitan community. *Am J Chron Dis* 37:609–615.
6. Kimball, A. M., S. B. Thacker, and M. E. Levy. 1980. Shigella surveillance in a large metropolitan area: assessment of a passive reporting system. *Am J Public Health* 70:164–166.
7. Vogt, R. L., D. Larue, D. N. Klaucke, D. A. Jillson. 1983. Comparison of active and passive surveillance systems of primary care providers for hepatitis, measles, rubella and salmonellosis in Vermont. *Am J Public Health* 73:795–797.

8. Thacker, S. B., S. Redmond, R. Rothenberg et al. 1986. A controlled trial of disease surveillance strategies. *Am J Prev Med* 2:345–350.
9. Alter, M. J., M. A. Hadler et al. 1987. The effect of underreporting on the apparent incidence and epidemiology of acute viral hepatitis. *Am J Epidemiol* 125:133,139.
10. Rosenberg, M. L. 1977. Shigella surveillance in the United States, 1975. *J Infect Dis* 136:458–459.
11. Marks, J. S., G. C. Hogelin, and E. M. Gentry et al. 1985. The behavioral risk factor surveys: I. State-specific prevalence estimates of behavioral risk factors. *Am J Prev Med* 1:1–8.
12. Graitcer, P. L., and A. H. Burton. 1987. The epidemiologic surveillance project: a computer-based system for disease surveillance. *Am J Prev Med* 3:123–127.

4

Disease Surveillance at the State and Local Levels

Gregory R. Istre

Public health surveillance was originally developed to control communicable or infectious diseases. As the tools of prevention have been expanded from quarantine to vaccinations, antibiotic prophylaxis and treatment, hygiene measures, and organized disease prevention programs, so the role of public health surveillance has grown to include disease control and prevention, the evaluation of public health practices, and the anticipation of health problems and health resource needs. In recent years, its role has been expanded to include other important public health problems, including injuries, chronic diseases, environmental exposures, and occupational diseases. For all of these problems, the authority for reporting and surveillance rests with state and local health departments through state laws and regulations.

Disease surveillance at the national, state, and local levels helps to define populations of people affected by a disease, to determine trends in the occurrence of disease, to explain the natural history of disease and changes in the etiologic agent, and to identify target groups for disease prevention and control activities.[1] It is only at the state and local levels, however, where a major role of surveillance is to expeditiously implement interventions to prevent the spread of disease. These interventions may involve the use of prophylactic antibiotics, such as rifampin for meningococcal exposure; passive immunization, such as immune globulin for hepatitis A exposure; active immunization, such as measles vaccine; or education, such as the role of personal cleanliness as a defense against the spread of shigella. At this level, prevention is usually focused on the individual or on small groups, such as household contacts, day-care classrooms, and so forth; it may occasionally involve a community, as in the case of

42

spraying for mosquito control or education about mosquito avoidance, in response to an outbreak of arboviral encephalitis. Because state and local health departments have the ability and the mandate to invoke intervention activities, they need more detailed information about cases, such as names, addresses, telephone numbers, and other locating information, in order to effectively perform disease control activities.

In addition, most of the feedback to individuals who report cases of disease occurs at the state and local levels. This includes feedback to physicians, laboratories, infection control practitioners, and so forth, and may take the form of personal contact to obtain further information about cases or to give feedback as a result of an investigation, or it may take the form of more formal feedback such as newsletters, reports, or other special mailings. This feedback is an important factor in maintaining public health surveillance.[2-4]

Almost all of the data reported from the National Notifiable Disease Surveillance System, which manages the routine analysis of nationally reportable diseases, is collected initially at the state or local level. In many ways, the contact with the reporting sources (physicians, laboratories, and infection control practitioners) by state and local personnel, and the disease intervention activities which are initiated as a result of a report, fosters the continued surveillance for these nationally notifiable diseases. The rapport which is established at the state and local levels between public health personnel and reporting sources ultimately determines the success of national disease surveillance activities. Ironically, little has been written about the mechanism and maintenance of such surveillance systems at the state and local levels.

MECHANISM AND MAINTENANCE OF SURVEILLANCE SYSTEMS

"Reporting" Does Not Equal "Surveillance"

There is a common misconception that designating a disease or condition as officially "reportable" is the same as conducting surveillance for that disease or condition. Nothing could be further from the truth. Officially designating a disease or condition as reportable is a one-time activity that simply provides a framework for surveillance. The actual surveillance for that disease or condition is an ongoing, dynamic activity that requires frequent, sustained interaction with reporting sources. A surveillance system for any disease requires nurturing, in the form of feedback and follow-up of reported cases. Although most diseases or conditions for which

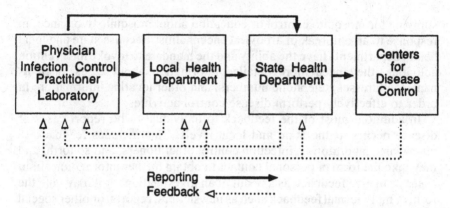

FIGURE 4-1.   Schematic diagram of the reporting–feedback loop that comprises public health surveillance systems. (Adapted from Klauce et al. 1988. *MMWR* 37(S-5):1–18.)

there is ongoing surveillance are also officially reportable, the latter is not necessary for the former to take place.

There are several characteristics that are generally applicable to successful surveillance programs. First, they involve disease or conditions which are perceived to be of public health importance. For example, surveillance for meningococcal disease, which is commonly considered to be of substantial public health importance, is more successful than that for aseptic meningitis, which is probably considered less important. Second, health care personnel, who are responsible for reporting, understand the importance of follow-up of cases, such as determining whether a case of hepatitis A is related to a day-care center. Third, there is an understanding of the reporting system, there is regular feedback, and in some program activities, there are incentives for reporting.

The Surveillance–Feedback Loop

A prototypical view of surveillance involves the several steps in the process of case reporting, data analysis, and feedback to reporting sources, as described by the Centers for Disease Control (CDC)[5] (see Figure 4-1).

For most diseases for which surveillance is conducted at a state or local level, the initial recognition and reporting occurs from physicians, diagnostic laboratories, infection control practitioners (ICPs), or institutions such as day-care centers, prisons, or long-term care facilities. Generally, physicians and laboratories are legally required to report certain diseases or conditions;[6, 7] in some states, certain institutions are also legally required to report. ICPs frequently are responsible for reporting cases of reportable diseases in hospitalized persons, a duty often delegated to them by physicians and directors of hospital-based laboratories through infection control committees or other bodies.

Disease reports are then made to either the state or local health department, depending on the guidelines established in that state. It is here that the first step in the feedback process begins; cases are followed up to assure that appropriate preventive intervention takes place. At this level the person who is designated to perform the follow-up, such as a public health nurse or a disease intervention specialist, frequently must contact the physician who managed the case, or the ICP who has access to the patient's medical record, to obtain information about the treatment that was given or whether prophylaxis was begun, if appropriate for the disease. At this point the physician may learn that the reported case is part of an outbreak; for example, a day care–associated shigella outbreak. This process, with the clear message that follow-up is being done, probably reinforces to physicians and ICPs the importance of reporting.[8] It seems likely that more timely and appropriate follow-up by public health agencies results in a higher rate of compliance with reporting, although there is little published information to support this contention.

At the state health department, patient identifying information is removed from records before being forwarded weekly to the CDC. Analysis of surveillance data takes place at the state health departments, the CDC, and in some large county and city health departments. At all levels, analysis identifies trends, affected populations, and potential target groups for disease prevention activities.[1] At the state and local levels, further attempts are usually made to recognize clusters of diseases or settings that enhance infection transmission risks, such as hepatitis A in foodhandlers and day-care attendees, or their families.

Feedback to reporting sources occurs at all levels in the system. As mentioned above, county or state health department personnel, such as nurses, disease intervention specialists, and epidemiologists often provide timely feedback during the investigation of the case. In addition, most state and several city and county health departments produce newsletters on a regular basis that provide disease-related statistics and analytic descriptions of these data, which are sent to the sources of reports.[1, 2, 8, 9] There also may be advisory information sent to physicians, ICPs, laboratories, and other potential reporting sources to alert them to an urgent problem, such as a measles outbreak or cases of a new disease or syndrome, as recently happened with the emergence of the eosinophilia-myalgia syndrome.[10] At the national level, the CDC provides feedback on a weekly basis to reporting sources as well as county, city, and state health departments through the *Morbidity and Mortality Weekly Report (MMWR)* and other special mailings.[1, 3] This combination of sources of timely feedback completes the surveillance loop and reinforces the dynamic properties of the surveillance system.[2]

Mandatory Reporting as a Framework for Surveillance

The recommendations for diseases to be included in the National Notifiable Disease Surveillance System are made by the U.S. Council of State and Territorial Epidemiologists (CSTE) at its annual meeting.[3] These recommendations are not legally binding in any state, and there are several diseases that are included in the National Notifiable Disease System that may not be legally reportable in several states.[6]

All states have some mandatory reporting requirements, although there are variations in the lists of diseases that are legally reportable for each state.[6, 7] A list of diseases and conditions that are legally reportable in most states can be found in Table 4-1. The legal mechanism for making a disease or condition reportable at the state level varies from state to state. In some states, diseases can be added to the list of those that are legally reportable only by the state legislature through changes or additions to state statutes or codes. In some states, a state board of health may determine which diseases are legally reportable, and in others the state health officer or commissioner would mandate that certain diseases be legally reportable.[6]

In fact, even with the force of law, the reporting of diseases is almost never enforced. A major benefit of making a disease or condition reportable may be the provision of a mechanism by which a physician may share important information about a patient with a reportable disease, within the context of patient–physician confidentiality, for the protection of the public health. In this sense, the advantage of making a disease legally reportable may lie in the removal of at least one barrier that may interfere with good surveillance: a concern for patient confidentiality.

Effective, ongoing surveillance can be maintained for certain diseases without mandatory reporting. Several states have sentinel systems for influenza-like illness surveillance, which often involves the reporting of numbers of cases seen by these sentinel physicians, without personal identifiers being used, as outlined below.

Types of Surveillance

Surveillance programs can be divided into four general categories: passive, active, sentinel, and special systems. The most commonly practiced dis-

TABLE 4-1   Diseases and Conditions That Are Reportable in a Majority[1] of States

Disease/Condition	Number of States and Territories[2] with Required Reporting	Disease/Condition	Number of States and Territories[2] with Required Reporting
AIDS	56	Malaria	56
Amebiasis	51	Measles	56
Anthrax	54	Meningitis, aseptic	43
Botulism	53	Meningitis, bacterial	30
Brucellosis	56	Meningococcal Disease	51
Campylobacteriosis	44	Mumps	55
Chancroid	43	Outbreaks	33
Chickenpox–Zoster	33	Pertussis	56
Chlamydia	34	Plague	49
Cholera	54	Poliomyelitis	56
Diphtheria	56	Psittacosis	52
Encephalitis	52	Rabies	54
Food-associated Illness	45	Reye Syndrome	48
Giardiasis	46	Rocky Mt. Spotted Fever	47
Gonorrhea	56	Rubella	55
Granuloma inguinale	36	Rubella, congenital	43
Hemophilus influenzae; invasive	43	Salmonellosis	53
		Shigellosis	53
Hepatitis A	50	Syphilis	56
Hepatitis B	50	Tetanus	56
Hepatitis Non-A, Non-B	44	Toxic Shock Syndrome	43
Hepatitis Unspecified	38	Trichinosis	53
Legionellosis	48	Tuberculosis	56
Leprosy	47	Tularemia	50
Leptospirosis	51	Typhoid Fever	55
Lyme Disease	32	Typhus	30
Lymphogranuloma venereum	38	Yellow Fever	43

[1] At least 30 states.
[2] Includes all the states, the District of Columbia, Puerto Rico, Guam, American Samoa, the Northern Mariana Islands, and the U.S. Virgin Islands.
SOURCE: Chorba et al. 1989. *JAMA* 262:3018–3026.

ease surveillance at state and local health departments involves passive surveillance, which generally uses standardized reporting cards or forms that are distributed in batches to clinics, hospitals, laboratories, and other health care settings.[11, 12] This type of system usually targets physicians, laboratories, or ICPs. It is referred to as a passive system because no action is taken unless completed reports are received by the public health agency. Completeness of reporting is usually lowest for passive systems, but such systems tend to be the least expensive to maintain. Heightened passive surveillance involves additional stimuli to generate reports, such as actions taken during some outbreaks or other occurrences of disease.

Active surveillance involves an ongoing search for cases. This may involve regular contacts with key reporting sources, such as telephone calls to physicians or laboratories, or a frequent review of data that may include cases of a specific condition, such as a review of laboratory logs for certain bacterial isolates, or a review of admissions to burn units to identify severely burned individuals. The frequency of contact may vary with the condition. Active systems may have high levels of completeness of reporting, but are usually much more expensive to maintain. There are conflicting reports in the literature about the cost-effectiveness of active surveillance.[13-15]

Sentinel systems involve the use of a sample of providers (most generally, a sample of physician practices or emergency rooms) to identify trends in diseases that occur at relatively high frequency. For example, sentinel surveillance systems, such as those for influenza, provide timely information about trends in influenza-like illness activity, and are useful in obtaining information about strains of influenza that may be circulating in a community, if there is a laboratory-based component to the surveillance. Sentinel systems are less useful in surveillance for diseases that necessitate follow-up to intervene to prevent their spread, such as hepatitis A or meningococcal infections, since more complete reporting and patient identifying information are important in effectively preventing these diseases.[16]

Special systems have been found to be useful for certain types of surveillance activities. For example, the Behavioral Risk Factor Surveillance (BRFS) involves administering a questionnaire via telephone to a random sample of individuals on an ongoing basis to identify trends in behaviors that affect health risk. This system has been found to be useful in monitoring the impact of such activities as breast cancer screening with mammography, cervical cancer screening with pap smears, the use of smoke alarms in houses, and other health-related behaviors and practices.[17] In addition, several knowledge, attitude, and behavior (KAB) surveys have been useful in determining the impact of public health education, especially in the area of AIDS prevention education.[18]

Microbiologic surveys have been useful in determining the prevalence of vaccine-related serotypes and antibiotic resistance among persons with invasive pneumococcal infections,[19] the occurrence of cholera by systematically identifying whether *Vibrio cholera* is present in sewage,[20] and the change in antimicrobial susceptibility patterns among various bacteria.[21, 22] Another source, hospital discharge data, has been found to be quite useful in determining trends in hospitalization for a variety of diseases and

TABLE 4-2   Advantages and Disadvantages of Selected Reporting Sources

Source	Advantages	Disadvantages
Physicians	Only source for nonlaboratory diagnosed diseases that don't require hospitalization.	Generally low completeness of reporting for most diseases. Dependent upon compliance from a large proportion of physicians.
Laboratories	Higher level of completeness of reporting. Can identify nonhospitalized as well as hospitalized cases. May use single source from each laboratory.	Not useful for diseases for which there is no single diagnostic test. Entirely dependent upon physicians ordering the appropriate specimens and tests.
Infection Control Practitioners	High level of completeness of reporting. May use single source from each hospital. Useful for clinically diagnosed as well as lab-confirmed cases.	Only useful for hospitalized cases.
Specialty Units	High level of completeness. Usually involves fewer sources.	Only useful for cases that are referred to the unit. May be biased by referral patterns. Useful for a limited number of conditions.

conditions.[23] It is worth noting that the success of the special surveillance system, and virtually all of the sentinel surveillance systems, does not involve making the disease or condition legally reportable.

Sources of Surveillance Data

Among the many potential sources of surveillance reports, four are commonly used in disease surveillance systems at the state and local levels: physicians, laboratories, ICPs, and specialty units (see Table 4-2).

Surveillance for diseases, especially infectious diseases, is often equated with physician reporting. In fact, most reports of communicable diseases come from sources other than physicians.[11, 15] The major disadvantage of relying on physicians for disease surveillance is that physicians often do not remember to report cases that they diagnose, and are often too busy to complete report forms. Surveillance systems that rely on physician reporting generally have a lower completeness of reporting than do other reporting sources.[11] Nevertheless, physicians may be the only available source for certain diseases for which the diagnosis may be made only on clinical grounds and without a specific laboratory test, such as toxic shock syndrome, especially for those cases who are not hospitalized.

Clinical laboratories are useful for the surveillance of certain diseases for which there is a definitive laboratory test, such as stool culture for diagnosis of salmonella, shigella, or campylobacter infection. However, laboratory-based surveillance has little or no role in surveillance for diseases for which there is no such definitive laboratory test, such as toxic shock syndrome, Kawasaki syndrome, tetanus, and so forth. Some laboratory-based, passive surveillance systems have had documented sensitivities as high as 80 percent for shigella,[11] but others have shown completeness of reporting which varies from 30 to 62 percent.[12, 24] An advantage of laboratory-based surveillance is that it includes cases of illness diagnosed in outpatients as well as those diagnosed in hospitalized persons. This type of surveillance is almost entirely dependent upon the practicing physician obtaining the appropriate specimen, since without these specimens there could be no surveillance. For example, Rosenberg et al. estimated that fewer than one-third of persons with shigellosis seen by a physician had stool specimens obtained for culture.[25]

ICPs tend to provide a substantial proportion of reports of infectious diseases.[15] ICPs are generally more oriented toward identifying cases of reportable diseases, since their jobs involve seeing that proper infection control practices are followed in the hospital setting. In most hospitals, the ICP is given the responsibility for reporting diseases to public health authorities by the physicians on staff at that hospital. The major drawback to ICP-based reporting is that this system is mainly useful for cases of diseases in hospitalized persons, and generally not as useful for cases occurring in outpatients.

Specialty units have been used with success to monitor conditions such as burns and spinal cord injuries. One surveillance system based in local and regional burn units has found very high completeness of reporting of hospitalized burn injuries.[26] In another setting, spinal cord rehabilitative centers have been used successfully statewide to monitor spinal cord injuries.[27] Although these specialty units may generate high levels of completeness of reporting, they are only useful in identifying cases that have been referred to these units, which in turn may represent only a small portion of the total cases, depending on referral patterns in that geographic area.

Generally, the most successful surveillance systems at the state and local levels involve multiple sources of reporting, including physicians, laboratories, and ICPs.[28, 29] Surveillance systems tend to be more complete if they are active rather than passive, and if they rely on laboratories, ICPs, or multiple sources of reports. In many states, certain diseases are legally reportable by both physicians and laboratories, which serves to increase the completeness of such reporting. It is probable that only through multiple sources can one expect a high degree of completeness of reporting/surveillance for a disease or condition which includes clinically diagnosed as well as laboratory-confirmed cases, and hospitalized as well as nonhospitalized cases.

Problems with Surveillance

Some problems that can interfere with the success of a surveillance system include lack of awareness, lack of understanding of the importance of surveillance, lack of feedback, and the presence of a complicated and difficult system. It is a most basic fact that if the sources of the report (i.e., physicians, laboratories, ICPs) are not notified that a disease or condition is reportable, the surveillance system will be doomed to fail. In addition, since there are very few instances of adverse legal consequences for nonreporting, the success of surveillance depends upon the goodwill between the state and local health departments and the sources of reports. Even if physicians, laboratories, and ICPs are aware that a given disease or condition is reportable, surveillance will suffer if it is perceived that little or nothing is done with the reports and if there is little or no feedback about them.[30] For example, Vogt et al. found that only 6 percent of cases of aseptic meningitis that were found by a review of hospital discharge data in Vermont had been reported.[31] It is likely that this was due, at least in part, to a correct perception by physicians, laboratories, and ICPs that little or no follow-up for cases of aseptic meningitis is done, that there are no public health preventive measures available to close contacts of cases, and thus that these reports result in no tangible benefit to public health.

Evaluation

Evaluation of surveillance systems is a task that should be built into each system. Such evaluation is important in ensuring that the surveillance systems operate efficiently and that only important problems are under surveillance.[5, 32] Although there are few reports in the literature that evaluate different surveillance systems, the CDC has recently published guidelines for such an evaluation.[5]

Confidentiality, Access, and Protection

All states have some degree of protection of confidentiality for persons whose names are reported to state and local health departments.[33] The issues surrounding the AIDS and HIV epidemic have heightened concerns for confidentiality and led to tighter controls and security measures for the protection of public health surveillance data.[34] Nevertheless, the statutes that address confidentiality vary from state to state, making it essential that public health personnel be knowledgeable about the details of the statutes for their state. It is common for physicians to be concerned about the release of potentially sensitive information to public health personnel, such as sexual orientation or illicit drug use, until they are familiar with the legal protections that exist for the patient to prevent the information from being divulged to others, and for the physicians, to protect themselves from litigation.

Further, some states have legal protection for institutions such as hospitals to share information for the protection of the public health. An outbreak of hospital-acquired infections, for example, is almost always a sensitive issue for the hospital involved. In at least one state, a statute protects reports of such problems, which are made to the state health department "for the purpose of reducing morbidity and mortality," from use in legal action against that institution.[35]

Public health departments have a long history of being able to maintain and protect the confidentiality of persons with communicable diseases whose names have been reported to them, a characteristic which has continued through the AIDS epidemic.[36] Confidentiality has been an essential element of successful surveillance systems and comprehensive disease control programs, and likely will continue to be so for the foreseeable future.

CONCLUSION

State and local health departments play a vital role in the dynamic process that is required to maintain effective public health surveillance. As surveillance continues to expand into noncommunicable disease areas such as chronic diseases, environmental health, and injuries, it is likely that this role will continue, if not become even more prominent. The issues of feedback, mandatory reporting, confidentiality, and evaluation likely will continue to be important issues in public health surveillance.

ACKNOWLEDGMENTS

The author appreciates the help of Genny Van Dorn in the preparation of the manuscript, and the thoughtful reviews of Jeffrey P. Davis, M.D.; Richard L. Vogt, M.D.; and John R. Harkess, M.D.

Notes
1. Thacker, S. B., K. Choi, and P. S. Brachman. 1983. The surveillance of infectious diseases. *JAMA* 249:1181–1185.
2. Langmuir, A. D. 1963. The surveillance of communicable diseases of national importance. *NEJM* 268:182–192.
3. Thacker, S. B., R. L. Berkelman, and D. F. Stroup. 1989. The science of public health surveillance. *J Pub Health Pol* 10:187–203.
4. Thacker, S. B., and R. L. Berkelman. 1988. Public health surveillance in the United States. *Epidemiol Rev* 10:164–189.
5. Klaucke, D. N., J. W. Buehler, S. B. Thacker et al. 1988. Guidelines for evaluating surveillance systems. *MMWR* 37(S-5):1–17.
6. Chorba, T. L., R. L. Berkelman, S. K. Safford, N. P. Gibbs, and H. F. Hull. 1989. Mandatory reporting of infectious diseases by clinicians. *JAMA* 262:3018–3026.
7. Freund, E., P. J. Seligman, T. L. Chorba, S. K. Safford, J. G. Drachman, and H. F. Hull. 1989. Mandatory reporting of occupational diseases by clinicians. *JAMA* 262:3031–3044.
8. Schaffner, W., H. D. Scott, B. J. Rosenstein, and E. B. Byrne. 1971. Innovative communicable disease reporting. *HSMHA Health Rep* 86:431–436.
9. Weiss, B. P., M. A. Strassburg, and S. L. Fannin. 1988. Improving disease reporting in Los Angeles County: trial and results. *Public Health Rep* 103:415–421.
10. Centers for Disease Control. 1989. Eosinophilia-myalgia syndrome: New Mexico. *MMWR* 38:765–767.
11. Harkess, J. R., B. A. Gildon, P. W. Archer, and G. R. Istre. 1988. Is passive surveillance always insensitive: an evaluation of shigellosis surveillance in Oklahoma. *Am J Epidemiol* 128:878–881.
12. Kimball, A. M., S. B. Thacker, and M. E. Levy. 1980. Shigella surveillance in a large metropolitan area: assessment of a passive reporting system. *Am J Public Health* 70:164–166.
13. Vogt, R. L., D. LaRue, D. N. Klaucke, and D. A. Jillson. 1983. Comparison of an active and passive surveillance system of primary care providers for hepatitis, measles, rubella, and salmonellosis in Vermont. *Am J Public Health* 73:795–797.
14. Hinds, M. W., J. W. Skaggs, and G. H. Bergeisen. 1985. Benefit-cost analysis of active surveillance of primary care physicians for hepatitis A. *Am J Public Health* 75:176–177.
15. Thacker, S. B., S. Redmond, R. B. Rothenberg et al. 1986. A controlled trial of disease surveillance strategies. *Am J Prev Med* 2:345–350.
16. Gunn, R. A. 1984. Active surveillance at the local level for communicable disease reporting. *Am J Public Health* 74:85–86.
17. Marks, J. S., G. C. Hogelin, E. M. Gentry, J. T. Jones, K. L. Gaines, M. R. Forman, and F. L. Trowbridge. 1985. The behavioral risk factor surveys: 1. State-specific prevalence estimates of behavioral risk factors. *Am J Prev Med* 6:1–8.

18. Becker, M. H., and J. G. Joseph. 1988. AIDS and behavior changes to reduce risk: a review. *Am J Public Health* 78:394–410.
19. Istre, G. R., M. Tarpay, M. Anderson, A. Pryor, D. F. Welch, and R. Facklam. 1987. A population-based study of invasive pneumococcal disease in an area with high rate of relative resistance to penicillin. *J Infect Dis* 176:932–935.
20. Blake, P. A., D. T. Allegra, J. D. Snyder et al. 1980. Cholera: a possible endemic focus in the United States. *NEJM* 123:424–430.
21. MacDonald, K. L., M. L. Cohen, N. T. Hargrett-Bean, J. G. Wells, N. D. Puhr, S. F. Collin, and P. A. Blake. 1987. Changes in antimicrobial resistance of *Salmonella* isolated from humans in the United States. *JAMA* 258:1496–1499.
22. Istre, G. R., J. S. Conner, M. Glode, and R. S. Hopkins. 1984. Increasing ampicillin resistance rates in *Haemophilus influenzae* meningitis. *Am J Dis Children* 138:366–369.
23. National Center for Health Statistics. 1977. *Development of the Design of the NCHS Hospital Discharge Survey.* Washington, D.C.: GPO, 1977. (Vital and health statistics. Series 2, no. 39, (DHEW publication no. (HRA) 77-1199.)
24. Marier, R. 1977. The reporting of communicable diseases. *Am J Epidemiol* 105:587–590.
25. Rosenberg, M. J., E. J. Gangarosa, R. A. Pollard et al. 1977. Shigella surveillance in the United States. *J Infect Dis* 136:458–460.
26. Makintubee, S., G. R. Istre, R. Ikard, and D. Krous. Oct. 22–26, 1989. Surveillance for injuries: from data to prevention. Paper presented at the 117th Annual American Public Health Association Meeting, Chicago, Ill.
27. Makintubee, S., G. R. Istre, R. Ikard, and D. Krous. Sept. 17–20, 1989. Epidemiology of traumatic spinal cord injuries: findings of a prototype surveillance system and implications for prevention. Paper presented at the First World Conference on Accident and Injury Prevention, Stockholm, Sweden.
28. Murphy, T. V., M. T. Osterholm, L. M. Pierson et al. 1987. Prospective surveillance of *Haemophilus influenzae* type B disease in Dallas County, Texas, and in Minnesota. *Pediatrics* 79:173–180.
29. Istre, G. R., J. S. Conner, C. V. Broome et al: 1985. Risk factors for primary invasive *Haemophilus influenzae* disease: increased risk from day care attendance and school-aged household members. *Pediatrics* 106:190–195.
30. Handsfield, H. H. 1990. Old enemies: combating syphilis and gonorrhea in the 1990s. *JAMA* 264:1451–1452.
31. Vogt, R. L., S. W. Clark, and S. Kappel. 1986. Evaluation of The State Surveillance System Using Hospital Discharge Diagnoses, 1982–1983. *Am J Epidemiol* 123:197–198.
32. Orenstein, W. A., and T. H. Bernier. 1990. Surveillance: information for action. *Pediatric Clinics of North America* 37:709–734.
33. Vogt, R. L. Confidentiality: perspectives from state epidemiologists. In: *Proceedings of the 1989 Public Health Conference on Records and Statistics.* DHHS Publication No. (PHS) 90-1214.

34. Torres, C. G., M. E. Turner, J. R. Harkess, and G. R. Istre. In press. Security measures for AIDS and HIV data. *Am J Public Health.*
35. Oklahoma Statutes. 1981. Title 63, Section 1-1709.
36. Association of State and Territorial Health Officials. 1988. *Guide to Public Health Practice: AIDS Confidentiality and Anti-discrimination Principles.* Washington, D.C.: Public Health Foundation.

5

Surveillance in Developing Countries

Michael D. Malison

Surveillance systems provide essential information for designing, implementing, and evaluating disease prevention and control activities. In the developing world, surveillance data are often untimely, incomplete, unrepresentative, and generally of such poor quality that confidence in the entire system is undermined. The process is cyclical—poor-quality data are not in demand, and the lack of demand further reduces incentives to improve quality. The cycle continues until some state of equilibrium is reached at which supply equals demand. In many instances, this equilibrium is determined by the demand set, not by program managers or decision makers, but by the archivists whose primary goal is to compile data for the annual statistical yearbook.

What factors affect the quality of surveillance data in the developing world? More specifically, given the resource constraints that all developing countries face, are there ways to increase both the supply of and demand for surveillance data? To answer these questions, let us review some of the attributes shared by many surveillance systems in the developing world.

One of the most prevalent characteristics of surveillance systems in the developing world is that they attempt to collect too much information about too many diseases and conditions. As the list of reportable diseases grows longer and the number of questions on each report form multiplies, the goal of surveillance grows more and more obscure. Highly endemic diseases or conditions can also overburden the system if reporting lacks specificity. For example, surveillance for gastroenteritis and malaria, rather than overwhelming the system, could be focused more specifically on the targets of prevention programs such as diarrhea with dehydration

56

or cerebral malaria. In addition to the volume of data surveillance systems are asked to collect, another characteristic of surveillance systems in the developing world is the lack of uniformity and the complexity of forms and administrative procedures that are required to report. This often results in confusion about who is supposed to report what, on which form, and to whom. Local health facility staff in most developing countries also have little or no idea of how surveillance data are used and generally do not see surveillance as meeting any of their managerial or programmatic needs. Lastly, surveillance data in the developing world are usually aggregated and tabulated, but are seldom analyzed or interpreted for the specific purpose of extracting information needed for public health practice. While the above description probably depicts a worst-case scenario, it illustrates the range and complexity of issues that affect the quality of surveillance data in the developing world. Let us now look at the process of surveillance and identify which components can be strengthened to make the system more efficient and useful.

DATA COLLECTION

To improve the quality of data collection, it is important to have an understanding of who reports, what skills are required to report, and what motivates individuals to report.

Responsibility for reporting in developing countries is often vague and diffuse. Physicians often feel it should be the nurses who report, and nurses complain that they do not have the authority to make an official diagnosis. The reluctance to accept responsibility for reporting may actually indicate a more fundamental problem: the need to limit personal liability for reporting in cultures where responsibility is often synonymous with culpability. Such problems are deep-rooted and take time to solve. The important point to get across is that the purpose of clarifying the responsibility for reporting is simply to ensure that surveillance is considered a routine activity and becomes part of someone's job description. It is not intended to make it easier to identify those persons who either report too much or too little.

Once it is clear who reports, the next question to address is whether these persons know what, how, and to whom to report. The lack of this specific information is perhaps the most common cause of underreporting. Such training, however, can be expensive, disruptive, and misused as a perquisite resulting in the training of inappropriate persons. A simpler and less costly alternative is to use the report form itself as a job-aid. If the list of reportable diseases is restricted to only those that are essential, and only essential information is requested about each case, it is often possible to print the list of reportable diseases directly on the form along with simple clinical case definitions. Surveillance case definitions that are provisional and based on clinical rather than laboratory criteria are an important concept to stress in the developing world, where undue concern over the correctness and finality of the diagnosis often impedes reporting. Preaddressed, franked forms can also simplify reporting and eliminate confusion about how and to whom reports should be sent. Obviously, adequate supplies of forms must be available at every reporting site for this approach to work.

In addition to catch-up strategies that provide essential information to existing health workers, information about surveillance should also be incorporated into preservice training programs, such as those in schools of medicine, nursing, and public health. Modifications to the curricula should be reinforced by including specific questions on surveillance in national examinations for professional licensure.

The final question of what motivates persons to report is perhaps the most difficult to address. One of the most common approaches used to stimulate reporting is the threat of punishment for failing to comply. In many instances, penalties for not reporting are incorporated into public health laws. In practice, such schemes are usually ineffective because they are impossible to enforce. Far more important are the disincentives for reporting—an unintentional attribute of many surveillance systems—which include the requirement to complete multiple forms for different diseases, the request for an excessive amount of information on each form, and the fear of being held personally liable for the occurrence of those diseases which one reports. Such disincentives affect both the quality and quantity of data reported. Ideally, report forms should be available in every facility where large numbers of patients are seen, the forms should be simple to complete (taking no more than a few minutes per form), and there should be one form for all reportable diseases. The more information the system tries to collect and the more complicated the procedures for reporting, the less motivation there is to report.

Besides minimizing disincentives for reporting, there are a number of ways to encourage reporting through more positive means. The key is to identify ways to make those who report "shareholders" in the surveillance system; in other words, those who initiate reports must realize a tangible benefit for doing so. The more proximate and tangible the benefit, the more likely persons are to report. In the waning days of the smallpox eradication program, for example, an actual cash reward was offered to stimulate reports of suspect cases. While such incentives are impractical on a broad scale, they illustrate the point.

Perhaps the best way to develop a strategy to stimulate reporting is to capitalize on preexisting local information needs. For example, most inpatient facilities have a strong interest in knowing how many patients they see by disease category or service. From their perspective, this information can be applied to better allocate resources and perhaps justify requests for budget increases. By understanding these needs, it should be possible to design a facility-based data collection system that serves the needs of both the surveillance system and the local facilities.

Another type of motivational tool for stimulating reporting is the epidemiologic bulletin or newsletter. Such publications are vehicles for disseminating information about surveillance, and can also serve as a forum for providing credit to those who have made an exceptional contribution, such as reporting an outbreak or finding creative ways to solve difficult problems. Feedback is an essential part of the surveillance loop and plays a vital role in motivating persons to report.

ANALYSIS AND INTERPRETATION

Once data are collected, they must be analyzed and interpreted in order to be meaningfully applied to disease prevention and control activities. In many developing countries, data are tabulated and aggregated by demographic categories, but there the process often ends. Ministries of health in the developing world are notoriously deficient in manpower with the basic skills needed to analyze, interpret, and apply the output of the surveillance system to the practice of public health. Epidemiologists are not necessarily in short supply in the developing world, but are most often employed by universities, not ministries of health. The reasons for this have to do with incentives; as faculty members, epidemiologists enjoy more prestige, are usually better paid, and have more opportunities to do research and publish than they would as employees of the ministry. The incentive systems of universities reward those who conduct original research and publish, not those who engage in the practice of public health offering their services to the ministry to analyze and interpret surveillance data. The disparity between the products of university-based research and the day-to-day needs of ministries of health in the developing world has grown so apparent in recent years that the World Health Organization (WHO) was recently compelled to pass a resolution calling for member countries to develop strategies to expand the use of epidemiology to ensure that Health for All by the Year 2000 objectives are met.[1] But how can this best be achieved? While this question is currently the topic of much debate, it is worth noting the progress that has been made in this area over the past decade.

Since 1980, the Southeast Asia Regional Office (SEARO) of WHO has been working with the U.S. Centers for Disease Control and the governments of Thailand and Indonesia to implement Field Epidemiology Training Programs (FETPs). Personnel from these programs are responsible for analyzing and interpreting surveillance data and applying it to disease prevention and control activities. Besides increasing the demand for surveillance data, the FETPs are actively involved in the feedback loop assisting local staff in conducting outbreak investigations and publishing their findings in epidemiologic bulletins. With a view to the future, trainees in today's FETPs are tomorrow's decision makers, learning first-hand the power of information as a tool for motivating persons and effecting change. By 1990, there were seven FETPs in three of the six WHO regions.[4, 5] To date, these programs have trained more than 100 epidemiologists, 98 percent of whom are still employed by their ministries of health.[5] Two new FETPs are now under development in collaboration with WHO's Western Pacific Regional Office (WPRO) and are expected to become operational in 1992.

SUMMARY AND CONCLUSIONS

Surveillance systems in the developing world are often overburdened by trying to collect too much information about too many diseases. As the system becomes less and less efficient, the quality of the data deteriorates and the goal of surveillance is lost. Factors that contribute to inefficiency include poorly defined responsibility for reporting, lack of knowledge about what and how to report, and the absence of meaningful incentives. Another factor that affects the demand for surveillance data is lack of epidemiologic manpower in most ministries of health. Improving surveillance in such settings is a challenging, but not impossible, task. One strategy that has been successful in a number of countries is the implementation of service-oriented, ministry-based Field Epidemiology Training Programs. Such programs offer an integrated approach to improving surveillance by increasing the demand for high-quality data, by applying the results of analysis to disease prevention and control activities, and by providing feedback to those involved in data collection. Disease surveillance is both necessary and practical in the developing world.

Notes
1. Pan American Health Organization. Epidemiology and the future of the world. *Epidemiol Bull* 1990;11(4):5.
2. World Health Organization. Field epidemiology training programme. *Wkly Epidemiol Rec* 1981; 56(7):49–52.

3. World Health Organization. Field epidemiology training for paramedical personnel. *Wkly Epidemiol Rec* 1987;62(36):265–268.
4. Malison, M. D., M. M. Dayrit, and K. Limpakarnjanarat. The Field Epidemiology Training Programmes. *Int J Epidemiol* 1989; 18(4):995–996.
5. Music, S. I., and M. G. Schultz. Field epidemiology training programs—new international health resources. *JAMA* 1990;263(24):3309–3311.

6

Hazard Surveillance

David H. Wegman

Epidemiologic surveillance is intended to provide early warnings that serve to guide timely intervention and prevention activities. By nature the systems utilize methods distinguished by their practicality, uniformity, and, frequently, their rapidity, rather than by their complete accuracy. The main purposes are to detect and follow changes in trends or distributions of health-related events in order to initiate control measures.

To consider the full potential of health surveillance it is worth looking closely at two common definitions. These are that surveillance is

> the ongoing, systematic collection, analysis, and interpretation of health data essential to the planning, implementation, and evaluation of public health practice, closely integrated with the timely dissemination of these data to those who need to know.[1]

and

> Surveillance implies the continuing observation of all aspects of the occurrence and spread of disease that are pertinent to its control.[2]

The use of the phrases "health data" and "all aspects of the occurrence and spread" provide the context to think as broadly as possible about health-"related" events, not just a disease, as objects for routine surveillance. This chapter is directed at considering the benefits to be derived from surveillance of hazards as a complement to surveillance of disease.

Hazard surveillance is the assessment of the occurrence of, distribution of, and the secular trends in levels of hazards (toxic chemical agents, physical agents, biomechanical stressors, as well as biologic agents) re-

62

sponsible for disease and injury. In a public health context, hazard surveillance identifies settings or individuals exposed to inappropriate or controllable levels of specific hazards.

There are already a number of familiar and important hazard surveillance activities which guide health policy. Several examples are illustrative:

1. Each summer, residents in urban areas who live near ocean beaches are informed of the safety of swimming at those beaches through published reports of coliform counts.
2. Health departments direct attention to the control of food poisoning outbreaks by their inspections of kitchens in public restaurants, which focus on a survey of hazardous conditions rather than cases of food poisoning.
3. In many large cities, published reports of daily variation in ozone levels are useful in guiding health protective behaviors for those who are susceptible to pulmonary disease.
4. Over a number of years, the monitoring of seat belt use and its association with injuries and fatalities in automotive accidents led manufacturers and the government to develop and introduce passive automotive restraints to protect the large number of nonusers.
5. A particularly effective hazard surveillance system follows the pattern of type-specific salmonella isolates reported by bacteriology laboratories nationwide. Routine examination of the results from these laboratory tests have proved highly successful in focusing early attention to point source outbreaks of salmonella epidemics.
6. A recent striking example of the impact of monitoring for hazards was the measurement of benzene contamination in a commercial bottled water. The finding led to a major product recall, and elimination of the source of benzene from the identified water supply.

What is it about hazard surveillance that makes it different from the better-known practice of disease surveillance?

BENEFITS OF HAZARD SURVEILLANCE

In public health, there are several potential benefits gained from hazard surveillance that expand on or complement those already provided by disease surveillance. These include: ease of measurement of the condition under surveillance, attention to the proper target of control, higher frequency of events, and avoidance of difficult issues of privacy.

Ease of Measurement

When considering infectious disease, the measurement (i.e., reliable diagnosis and reporting) of disease has been relatively straightforward. Routine reporting of measles, mumps, chickenpox, rubella, and so forth, has proven effective due, in large part, to the reliable diagnosis of the characteristic symptoms and disease course. As a result, the surveillance of childhood diseases has proven to be an effective public health tool, particularly in the targeting of efficient/effective immunization programs.

In contrast, the measurement of noninfectious disease, when applied to the purpose of disease surveillance, has generally been disappointing. This results from the fact that many noninfectious diseases have multiple causes, which often requires relatively specific linking of cause with disease before a report is useful for surveillance.

Rutstein et al. developed the concept of sentinel health events for surveillance by directing attention to diseases or conditions which, by their occurrence alone, provided evidence of a *preventable* disease, disability or death.[3] The list they developed included the common childhood infections as well as events such as maternal death. The underlying principle was that each condition, simply by its occurrence, provided enough evidence of preventable causes that public health action was indicated. However, when this concept was later adapted for use in recognizing and preventing occupational disease, the occurrence of the disease had to be conditioned on (linked to) the occurrence of appropriate exposure conditions as well.[4] For example, exposure to manganese is a recognized cause of Parkinson's disease. A public health effort to eliminate this cause of Parkinson's disease, however, would be poorly served by surveillance of the disease alone. Manganese is only one cause, and a proportionally small one compared with other, less clearly delineated causes. Thus, to accomplish the goal of preventing manganese-related Parkinson's disease would require surveillance of both disease and exposure simultaneously or possibly, as will be described, the surveillance of manganese exposure alone.

Proper Focus of Control

A second benefit from focusing on hazards for surveillance is that items under surveillance are also those to be targeted for primary prevention. For example, surveillance of the problem of asbestos-related lung cancer could focus on lung cancer in asbestos workers. However, a not insubstantial amount of lung cancer in such a population would be due to cigarette smoking either independent of, or interacting with, asbestos exposure. On the other hand, surveillance of asbestos exposure could provide information on the levels and patterns of exposure (jobs, processes, or industries) where the poorest exposure control exists. Then, even without an actual count of lung cancer cases, efforts to reduce or eliminate exposure would be appropriately targeted.

Frequency of Events

A further potential benefit from hazard surveillance is the much higher frequency of events. Exposures above a certain level can all be treated as an event on each occasion an exposure survey is undertaken. The higher level of detail regarding patterns and trends, along with the opportunity for limited, more targeted, investigations as needed, is in sharp contrast to that provided by the counts of a disease that occurs only once in an individual, and not even in all exposed individuals.

To take advantage of the higher frequency of hazard "events" compared with disease for surveillance, depends, however, on a central underlying assumption. Since hazard surveillance is directed at nondisease events, its use in guiding public health intervention requires that a clear exposure–outcome relationship has been established. With such a relationship established it can then be assumed that a reduction in exposure will result in reduced disease, obviating the need to document reduction in disease or adverse effects.

Although a quantitative exposure–response relationship is not necessary for hazard surveillance, its existence provides more effectvie guidance. For example, a well-described quantitative relationship between asbestos exposure and lung cancer allows an intervention to focus on the need to control exposures well below the level commonly associated with the disease. Once done, the disease can be assumed to be controlled without further documentation.

Note how the need for a clear exposure–disease relationship limits the potential applications of hazard surveillance. For example, in the case of repetitive trauma disorders (RTDs), epidemiologic studies have begun to show the increased prevalence of RTDs with awkward and highly repetitive motions. However, the development of good measures of these types of exposure and related exposure–outcome relationships is still in its infancy. At present, the lack of quantification of the exposure–disease associations, as well as only a crude understanding of the relative risk of different degrees of the "exposures," limits the creation of an effective hazard surveillance activity for RTDs.

Protection of Privacy

A particularly important advantage of hazard surveillance is that data collected for this purpose do not infringe on an individual's privacy. Confidentiality of medical records is not at risk and the possibility of stigmatizing an individual with a disease label is avoided. This is a particularly important advantage in industrial settings, where a person's job may be in jeopardy or a potential compensation claim may affect a physician's choice of diagnostic options.

Use of Existing Systems

There are a variety of existing systems that can be adapted for or directly utilized in hazard surveillance. This benefit of hazard surveillance parallels similar opportunities present for disease surveillance. Examples of ongoing collection of hazard information that already exist include such items as registries of toxic substance use or hazardous material discharges, registries for specific hazardous substances, and information collected for use in compliance activity. An example of this last activity, workplace monitoring information collected during regulatory inspections, is further described later in this chapter.

One unusual example of the potential recognized in an existing system concerns the possible use of routine corporate financial reports. Studies of the airline and trucking industries have suggested that financial stability relative to payroll size, proportion of expenses devoted to maintenance, and other similar factors predict future accident experience.[5] Specifically, as the proportion of funds used for repairs and maintenance decreases there is evidence that there is an increasing incidence of accidents within the trucking industry. A variety of financial indicators are used by accountants to routinely measure and predict the financial behavior and health of a business. These preliminary studies suggest that opportunity exists to examine similar economic features of a business as a hazard surveillance tool to predict safety and possibly health experience.

Using existing records rather than information from a system specifically designed for a surveillance function typically provides more general than detailed results. Their advantage, however, is that no new expenditures or reporting is required.

GENERAL ISSUES IN UNDERTAKING HAZARD SURVEILLANCE

The potential use of a hazard surveillance activity varies both by the latency period of the condition of interest and by a consideration of available alternatives.

Diseases of Long Latency

In the case of chronic conditions with long latency and without accessible, early indicators, hazard surveillance would appear to have special advantages over disease surveillance. For example, when disease surveillance is used for describing and tracking the patterns of cancer on a national, regional, or local basis, it is recognized that the information provided has limited value for primary prevention. Cancer surveillance results that provide the age, sex, race, and other general population characteristics for the cancer are useful in planning secondary prevention activity. Such findings may also have application in following trends in treatment or for identifying changing needs for acute and chronic medical care.

However, to the degree that the cancer has known environmental causes, disease surveillance alone is unlikely to be helpful in addressing these causes. Furthermore, unless the environmental causes do not vary by time and place, surveillance information on the spatial and temporal disease patterns are indicators only of historical, and not current risk.

By contrast, tracking the distribution of the known environmental causes of cancer provides evidence relevant to choices among intervention options directly related to the reduction or elimination of *current* risk (i.e., exposure). For those agents with well-described exposure–response relationships, the measure of reduced exposure following interventions represents an estimate of reduced future disease burden. It is important to be aware that this advantage of hazard surveillance is limited to those circumstances where an etiologic agent is known. As yet, many cancers have no known cause, and thus useful information for their control cannot be gained through hazard surveillance.

Conditions with Biomarkers

Conditions with long or short latency that have useful measures of biologic dose or subclinical effects provide a different opportunity. For example, surveillance directed at lead poisoning is quite different from that for cancer. In lead poisoning there is a biologic indicator of lead dose (blood lead levels) and there are several biologic indicators of early lead effects (e.g., fetal erythrocyte protoporphyrin [FEP]). Although it may take months or even years for cases of symptomatic lead poisoning to develop, either of these indicators could be used to provide early evidence of lead burden and of subclinical lead effects. Hazard surveillance efforts could be directed at measurements of lead in air, earth, house paint, or in blood. Disease surveillance could simultaneously be directed at recording cases of lead neurotoxicity, lead colic, or lead-induced anemias, or to monitoring blood levels of FEP.

Neither approach has as unique a public health advantage as was the case for hazard surveillance and environmental cancers. However, simultaneous surveillance directed both at patterns and changes in blood lead level (hazard surveillance) and at patterns and changes in FEP (disease surveillance) could be expected to have special advantages. Trends in blood lead could lead to early action on a job where legal limits are not exceeded but where surveillance documents a gradual increase in blood lead levels among employees, indicating exposure control failures. On the other hand, abnormal FEP measures may identify those experiencing effects from multiple sources of lead exposure not recognizable from blood lead levels alone.

Acute Exposure or Disease Events

A number of disease conditions are difficult to keep under useful surveillance because their latency period is so short. For example, it is difficult to imagine an effective surveillance (disease or hazard) for acute carbon monoxide poisoning or occupational asthma attacks due to chemical spills. In one sense, the events themselves are sentinels and require attention to their cause and consideration for future prevention. In both cases, recording the disease event would provide the desired sentinel information.

Hazard surveillance of carbon monoxide exposures around a gas-fired boiler, however, might indicate deteriorating conditions or intermittent peaks. These in turn might be traced to uncommon climatic conditions that help identify an impending leak of exhaust fumes. In the case of chemical spills, hazard surveillance could provide useful additional information of accidents "in search of a disease event." In this case the cause of the spills may be identified before anyone (or any susceptible person) is overexposed and suffers an asthma attack.

Agents Without Known Health Effects

In general the surveillance of hazards that are not yet associated with adverse health outcomes is unproductive. In this sense, hazard surveillance is not useful for hypothesis generation (one of the general goals of disease surveillance). However, the introduction of a new chemical or biologic agent may warrant surveillance simply to document, in appropriate detail, the level and distribution of exposure to the agent. While such information may not be immediately useful, it may serve an important function in the future when matched with information on disease as knowledge of health effects develops.

POTENTIAL USES FOR HAZARD SURVEILLANCE

In describing the nature, advantages, and limitations of hazard surveillance, a number of possible applications have been noted or can be inferred. The information from such systems can be seen as relevant to one of five objectives: to focus intervention actions, to set public health priorities, to provide macro- or microinformation on hazard prevalence, to determine appropriate resource allocation, and to contribute to epidemiologic studies.

Focusing Intervention Actions

Probably the most easily understood application of hazard surveillance is to contribute to focusing intervention actions. It should be evident that surveillance of any number of known hazards provides information on existing or developing hazardous conditions that need to be controlled. Further, depending on the level of detail available, the results from hazard surveillance can also contribute to identifying the likely reason(s) for the conditions. On another level, the careful use of hazard surveillance information can detect early evidence of a system failure and call attention to the need for improved controls (or repairs) before any excess exposures or diseases are actually experienced. Finally, data from such efforts can also provide evidence on whether there is need for new or revised regulation of the hazard.

Program Planning

In addition to directing specific intervention efforts, a broader use of hazard surveillance data is for program planning. For example, national or statewide information on the distribution of elevated lead levels in air samples stratified by either industry and job or the community should prove useful in determining how to plan general compliance activity. Comparative information of this type for several different exposures would further guide the placement of priorities with respect to the most important agents. The cumulative risk associated with elevations in several different exposures in the same location (for example, a particular industry) may call attention to a public health need not otherwise evident. Finally, matching this type of exposure information with exposure–response models for the relevant diseases has been suggested as a means to estimate disease burden.[6] In contrast to the recognized severe underreporting of occupational disease,[7] for example, the projected disease-specific burdens could be estimated and changes in the estimates can be tracked.

Levels of Focus

Exposure measurements can be made frequently, and standard methods allow for their collection in a variety of places by different personnel using established valid procedures. As a result there is detail potentially available at many different organizational levels that provides the opportunity for a number of different levels of surveillance. This flexibility permits a focus on a nation, a city, an industry, a plant, or even a job. With this flexibility surveillance can be targeted, adjusted as needed, and relatively easily revised and refined as new information becomes available or as problems go out of or come under control.

Resource Allocation

It has already been mentioned that hazard surveillance analyses provide the basis for compliance or intervention planning. A further application to resource allocation would be to use these data to estimate the need for different health services. Knowing the number and types of certain exposure events would be a valuable asset to health care providers in planning a community's clinical services for orthopedic, rehabilitation, and emergency medicine. Another less obvious use of the data would be to determine the need for worker or community education programs. These can then be targeted to apprise potentially affected individuals of the nature of hazards and the proper actions that are within an individual's control.

Epidemiologic Studies

Finally, hazard surveillance data should prove valuable to selecting and planning epidemiologic studies. Identification of areas or locations where specific types or levels of exposure exist is extremely valuable information when planning studies, which are often expensive and lengthy. An example of a first level of such information is the National Institute for Occupational Safety and Health, National Occupational Exposure Surveys—NOES.[8, 9] These surveys, carried out on a national population sample of workplaces, provide estimates of potential exposures in both full- and part-time occupations. Data derived from these have provided hitherto unavailable information on exposures in a variety of industries, aiding investigators in targeting potential study sites. Hazard surveillance activity that provided exposure information might prove useful in carrying out such studies as well.

EXAMPLES OF HAZARD SURVEILLANCE

The remainder of this chapter is devoted to providing examples of the uses of hazard surveillance.

Carcinogen Registry (Finland)

In 1979 Finland began to require national reporting of the use of 50 different carcinogens in industry. Reports were received from throughout the nation and the trends over the first seven years of surveillance were reported in 1988.[10] The results provided valuable information on potential exposure to the different carcinogens. For example, it was learned that 20,000 of 2.3 million workers were exposed to carcinogens at some time during the seven years, and that chromates, nickel and its organic compounds, and asbestos accounted for approximately two-thirds of all exposures. Analysis by occupation indicated that the highest proportion of the employed population with carcinogen exposures was metalplating and -coating workers (27.4 percent). Tracking all reports of exits from the registry suggested that 38 percent of removals resulted from substitution of noncarcinogens or the introduction of adequate exposure controls. One example was cited from the trend analysis which specifically documented the increasing substitution of a suspect carcinogen (hydrazine) by a noncarcinogen over the period of the survey. Although a number of limitations of the system are described in the report, the variety of potential applications of such a system is already compelling.

National Occupational Exposure Survey (NOES)

As noted, NIOSH carried out two National Occupational Exposure Surveys (NOES) ten years apart to estimate the number of workers and workplaces potentially exposed to each of a wide variety of hazardous exposures. One way in which data from these surveys have now become available is in the form of national and state maps showing distributions of any of the items surveyed. Examples, have been published[11] that show the pattern of workplace and worker exposures to formaldehyde. Taking these maps and superimposing them on maps of mortality for specific causes (e.g., nasal sinus cancer), provides the opportunity for simple ecologic examinations designed to generate hypotheses which can then be investigated by appropriate epidemiologic study.

A second application of these survey data has been to examine the change between the two surveys. For example, the proportion of facilities in which potential exposures were found to continuous noise without functioning controls were examined.[12] When examined by industry, little change was seen for general building contractors (92.5 to 88.4 percent), whereas a striking decrease was seen for chemicals and allied products (88.8 to 38.0 percent) and for miscellaneous repair services (81.1 to 21.2 percent). A variety of suggestions were made to explain the changes, including the passage of the Occupational Safety and Health Act, collective bargaining agreements, concerns with legal liability, and increased employee awareness.

Inspection (Exposure) Measures (OSHA)

The U.S. Occupational Safety and Health Administration (OSHA) has been inspecting workplaces to evaluate the adequacy of exposure controls for twenty years. For most of that time the data have been placed in a database, the Integrated Management Information System (OSHA/IMIS). These data can be examined in total for secular trends or according to a variety of specific strata, such as by job, by industry, or both. Although the data have the limitations of any data collected primarily for another purpose (the legal enforcement of exposure limits with potential emphasis on "worst-case situations") they appear to be reasonably representative of the likely exposure circumstances found in industry in general.[6]

Overall secular trends in selected cases have been published for the years 1979 to 1987.[13] These present some interesting findings. For asbestos, probably the most widely known of hazardous industrial agents, there is good evidence for largely successful controls. In contrast, although these years saw a decreasing number of samples collected for exposures to silica and lead, both continued to show a substantial number of overexposures. That these data suggest more attention—rather than less—should be directed to these exposures was clear. Interestingly, the data also showed that, despite reduced inspection measurements, the proportion of the number of exposure limit exceedences to the total number of samples in both cases has remained essentially constant. Such data should be highly instructive to OSHA when planning a compliance strategy related to these two substances.

Other uses of these data have been made. For example, a quantitative examination of the silica exposure levels for nine industries was performed, including a detailed look at jobs within each industry.[14] Exposure limit exceedences varied from 14 percent (aluminum foundries) to 73 percent (potteries). Within the potteries specific jobs were examined and the proportion with exceedences ranged from 0 percent (laborers) to 69 percent (sliphouse workers). A slightly different picture was revealed when examining the degree to which samples exceeded the exposure limit. For sliphouse workers exceedences were, on average, twice the exposure limit, while another job group, slip/glaze sprayers, had average exceedences of over eight times the limit. This level of detail should prove valuable to the management and workers employed in potteries as well as to government agencies responsible for regulating occupational exposures.

Related findings of interest were seen in a similar analysis of lead exposures.[15] The report concentrated on the six primary industries that were the focus of the U.S. lead exposure standard. A number of findings were similar in nature to those in the silica report. However, the analysis also revealed that there was unexpected widespread lead overexposure among painters in a variety of *machining* operations. Although painting with lead paint is a recognized hazardous job, these painters appear to have been forgotten, possibly because the predominant employment in the industry is machining, not painting. It is suggested that there may have been less vigilance than would have been the case if the industry were primarily involved in lead painting.

Priority Setting Using a National Database

It has already been shown how information from the NOES surveys by NIOSH and the OSHA/IMIS system might be used to suggest major priorities for regulators, company industrial hygienists, worker educators, and health authorities in general. One group of investigators has attempted to provide a way to integrate information from these resources so that industries or occupations can be evaluated for an estimated *total* hazardous exposure. Using the OSHA/IMIS data just described, in conjunction with information on the relative toxicity of each of the substances, an index was developed and applied to workforce-size data for specific industries and occupations in Los Angeles.[16] The results provided an estimate of the overall priorities for occupational exposure hazards in the county. This same approach was subsequently applied to all of New York state. The findings gave the first clear indication about the magnitude of the state's potential occupational disease problem and contributed significantly to a successful campaign to establish and fund statewide occupational health clinics.[17]

SUMMARY

This chapter was designed to identify the purpose of hazard surveillance, describe its benefits and some of its limitations, and to offer a variety of examples in which it has already provided useful public health information. It would be a mistake, however, to suggest that hazard surveillance was a panacea and should replace disease surveillance for noninfectious disease. In 1977 a NIOSH task force summarized the relative importance and interdependence of the two major types of surveillance.

The surveillance of hazards and diseases cannot proceed in isolation from each other. The successful characterization of the hazards associated with different industries or occupations, in conjunction with toxicological and medical information relating to the hazards, can suggest industries or occupational groups appropriate for epidemiologic surveillance.

Conversely, unusual health patterns in certain industries or occupations elucidated by surveillance of health effects will be more fully explained by surveillance of the potentially causative agents. A few disease entities, e.g., mesothelioma, are sufficiently cause-specific to diminish the need for hazard surveillance. Some agents are sufficiently effect-specific to make the task of illness surveillance relatively straightforward.

There remains, however, a vast middle ground where exposures are complex and symptoms diverse, which will yield only to the combined efforts of hazard and disease surveillance.[18]

Notes
1. Centers for Disease Control. Draft Policy Statement.
2. Benenson, A. S., ed. 1990. *Control of Communicable Disease in Man*. Washington, D.C.: American Public Health Association.
3. Rutstein, D. D., W. Berenberg, T. C. Chalmers, C. G. Child, A. P. Fishman, and E. B. Perrin. 1976. Measuring the quality of medical care: a clinical method. *NEJM* 294:582–588.
4. Rutstein, D. D., R. J. Mullan, T. M. Frazier et al. 1983. Sentinel health event (occupational): a basis for physician recognition and public health surveillance. *Am J Public Health* 73:1054–1062.
5. Bojolay, R. P. 1988. The effects of financial performance and deregulation in the trucking and airline industries on worker safety. Paper presented at the annual meeting of the American Public Health Association, Boston, Mass.
6. Froines, J. R., D. H. Wegman, and E. A. Eisen. 1989. Hazard surveillance in occupational disease. *Am J Public Health* 79(sup):26–31.
7. Pollac, E. S., and D. G. Keimig. 1987. *Counting Injuries and Illnesses in the Workplace: Proposals for a Better System*. Washington, D.C.: National Academy Press.
8. National Institute for Occupational Safety and Health. 1977. National occupational hazard survey. III. Survey analysis and supplemental tables. NIOSH pub. no. 780114. Order from national Technical Information Service, Springfield, Va. No. 1 PB-82-229-991/A99.
9. National Institute for Occupational Safety and Health. In press. National occupational exposure survey. I. Survey manual. Cincinnati, Ohio.
10. Alho, J., T. Kauppinen, and E. Sundquist. 1988. Use of exposure registration in the prevention of occupational cancer in Finland. *Am J Ind Med* 13:581–592.
11. Frazier, T. M., N. R. Lalich, and D. H. Pedersen. 1983. Uses of computer generated maps in occupational hazard and mortality surveillance. *Scand J Work Env Health* 9:148–154.
12. Seta, J. A., and D. S. Sundin. 1984. Trends of a decade—a perspective on occupational hazard surveillance 1970–1983. *MMWR* 34:15SS–24SS.

13. Frazier, Todd. Personal Communication.
14. Froines, J. R., D. H. Wegman, and C. A. Dellenbaugh. 1986. An approach to the characterization of silica exposure in U.S. industry. *Am J Ind Med* 10:345–361.
15. Froines, J. R., S. Baron, D. H. Wegman, and S. O'Rourke. 1990. Characterization of the airborne concentrations of lead in U.S. industry. *Am J Ind Med* 18:1–17.
16. Froines, J. R., C. A. Dellenbaugh, and D. H. Wegman. 1986. Occupational health surveillance: a means to identify work-related risks. *Am J Public Health* 76:1089–1096.
17. Landrigan, P. J., and S. B. Markowitz. 1987. Occupational disease in New York state: proposals for a statewide network of occupational disease diagnosis and prevention centers. New York: Environmental and Occupational Medicine Laboratory, Mount Sinai School of Medicine.
18. Sundin, D. S., D. H. Pedersen, and T. M. Frazier. 1986. Editorial: Occupational hazards and health surveillance. *Am J Public Health* 76:1083–1084.

7

Surveillance in the Control of Vaccine-Preventable Diseases*

Walter A. Orenstein and Roger H. Bernier

The United States Immunization Program is one of the most successful prevention programs in public health. Data from 1991 indicate that reductions of greater than 90 percent from peak reporting levels occurred for measles, mumps, rubella, congenital rubella syndrome (CRS), diphtheria, tetanus, pertussis, and polio (see Table 7-1). Most of the reductions are in the 98- to 99-percent range. This remarkable success is the result of the appropriate use of safe and effective vaccines. Critical to appropriate use is an information system that allows the measurement of health impact, the definition of target populations for vaccination, the evaluation of the impact of the vaccination program, and the detection of problems requiring alterations in vaccination strategies.

The information system consists of two components, surveillance and special studies or investigations. This chapter describes the role of surveillance in the management of immunization programs and the role of the clinician in assuring that adequate data are available.

GENERAL CONCEPTS OF SURVEILLANCE

Most persons equate surveillance with the monitoring of trends in the reporting of communicable diseases such as measles, polio, and so forth. With regard to immunization, however, surveillance also includes the

---

* Reprinted with permission from a previous publication, with minor changes, from *Pediatric Clinics of North America* 37:709–734. Philadelphia: W. B. Saunders Company, 1990.

TABLE 7-1   Comparison of Maximum and Current Morbidity Vaccine-Preventable Disease

	Maximum Cases (Year)	1991 (Prov.)	Percent Change
Diphtheria	206,939 (1921)	2	−99.99
Measles	894,134 (1941)	9,488	−98.94
Mumps[1]	152,209 (1968)	4,031	−97.35
Pertussis	265,269 (1934)	2,575	−99.03
Polio (paralytic)	21,269 (1952)	0	−100.00
Rubella[2]	57,686 (1969)	1,372	−97.62
CRS[3]	20,000 (1964–5)[2]	36	−99.82
Tetanus[4]	601 (1948)	49	−91.85

[1] First reportable in 1968
[2] First reportable in 1966
[3] First reportable in 1947
[4] Congenital rubella syndrome

monitoring of vaccine coverage and adverse events associated with vaccination.[1, 2] Recently, the Division of Immunization established a surveillance system to monitor lawsuits filed against manufacturers of diphtheria and tetanus toxoids and pertussis vaccine (DTP).[3] In contrast, one-time serosurveys or surveys of disease histories in a population are more appropriately classified as special studies.

Surveillance systems tend to generate incomplete data. For example, prior to the licensure of measles vaccines in 1963, approximately 400,000 to 500,000 cases were reported annually at a time when roughly 4,000,000 children were born each year. Since serologic and historical surveys indicated that virtually everyone was infected with measles virus by adulthood, approximately one birth cohort should have been infected annually at steady state conditions.[4] Thus, the 400,000 to 500,000 cases reported represented approximately 10 percent of the total cases occurring in the United States. A recent evaluation of surveillance of CRS shows a similar reporting efficiency.[5] Thus, surveillance data represent a sample. However, in contrast to the randomly chosen sample used in most research studies, the sample in surveillance data is selective and is influenced by a number of potential biases. For example, reports of pertussis cases tend to include persons with the most severe disease. Of the 4,728 cases reported to the Centers for Disease Control (CDC) between 1984 and 1985 for which data were available, 41 percent were hospitalized.[6] This contrasts sharply with community-based studies in which hospitalization rates generally are less than 10 percent.[7-9] Nevertheless, despite incompleteness and potential biases, surveillance data have been remarkably useful in serving the needs of public health programs.

SOURCES OF DATA

Surveillance information can come from a variety of sources, including health care providers, laboratories, hospital records, death certificates, and from a host of other persons such as school nurses.[10-13] Most surveillance systems rely upon case reports by physicians. This is particularly true for diseases with characteristic clinical symptoms and signs such as measles and mumps, where few cases are hospitalized and few attempts are made to confirm cases through the laboratory. Physician reporting has the advantage in that diagnoses are more likely to be accurate, since the report is made by someone skilled in differential diagnosis. It also offers the potential of more rapid reporting, since the notification can be made the day the case is initially seen. In contrast, when relying on school nurses, who may not be aware of the illness until the child returns to school, reports may be delayed. This can hamper control efforts if vaccination programs need to be started at the time of the first case. On the other hand, while school-nurse reporting may not be as specific as physician reporting, school-nurse reporting may be more sensitive, since many persons with measles may not seek medical care. Using information from both sources may be preferable to relying on a single source.

Laboratories and hospitals can be more useful for surveillance of diseases such as *Haemophilus influenzae* type b because most cases of invasive illness are both hospitalized and confirmed via the laboratory. Laboratory surveillance is also important in pertussis and rubella cases because of the difficulties in making the clinical diagnosis.

Mortality records are used for evaluating health impact and the characteristics of persons who die with a given disease. A special surveillance system that includes deaths registered in 121 U.S. cities each week is used to determine the existence of an epidemic of influenza by comparing the reported proportion of total deaths due to pneumonia and influenza with expected proportions based on nonepidemic years.[14]

Case Definitions

Epidemiologists tend to use standardized, uncomplicated case definitions in surveillance programs.[13, 15] These definitions may be difficult for clinicians to accept since they tend to greatly simplify the complex process used to arrive at a clinical diagnosis. For example, the current definition for a probable case of measles includes three terms: (1) generalized rash of ≥ 3 days duration; (2) fever (maximum temperature $\geq 101°F$, if measured); and (3) one of the following: (*a*) cough, (*b*) coryza, or (*c*) conjunctivitis.[16] The measles case definition is very sensitive in that it detects the majority of cases; however, it lacks specificity in that it includes many noncases. Nevertheless, this definition offers guidance in evaluating case reports and is useful for disease control purposes.

Case definitions vary with the goals of the surveillance system. For example, prior to beginning a vaccination program, or during its early phases, all physician reports are usually accepted (i.e., the case definition is physician diagnosis). However, as incidence decreases and a greater degree of disease control is achieved, individual cases are investigated by health department personnel, and case definitions tend to become more precise. For example, in some states, the case definition for measles will also require laboratory confirmation or epidemiologic linkage to another case meeting the same clinical criteria. Clinical information from reported suspected cases of poliomyelitis is now reviewed by a panel of three experts before being accepted as a case. These stricter definitions increase the predictive value positive of reported cases. The predictive value positive would normally fall as disease incidence decreases unless stricter definitions are used.

The appendix to this chapter lists the current case definitions used by the CDC for notifiable vaccine-preventable diseases.[17] Most of these definitions are based on clinical and epidemiologic experience; some have been evaluated for sensitivity and specificity during special investigations. For example, outbreak investigations in Wisconsin and Delaware revealed that a case definition for pertussis of cough for 14 or more days duration was 84 to 92 percent sensitive and 63 to 90 percent specific in the outbreak setting.[18]

The ideal sensitivity and specificity of case definitions depends upon the outcomes desired from surveillance. For controlling outbreaks, particularly during disease elimination and eradication, high sensitivity with rapid reporting becomes important for early action. For studies, such as vaccine efficacy evaluation, specificity assumes greater importance.[19]

Physician Reporting

Each state has a list of diseases that physicians, laboratories, and other health care providers are required to report by law.[10, 20] Usually the reporter is required to fill out a form or postcard. For some diseases, immediate notification via telephone is required. While the laws may provide for penalties such as suspension of a physician's license for failure to report, in practice such penalties are difficult to enforce.[21]

The Council of State and Territorial Epidemiologists (CSTE) in collaboration with the CDC develops the list of diseases that should be reported to the CDC. At the present time, among the vaccine-preventable diseases, cases of measles, mumps, rubella, CRS, diphtheria, tetanus, pertussis, and polio are officially reportable via state agencies and the District of Columbia on a weekly basis to the CDC. *Haemophilus influenzae* type b (Hib) has recently been added to the list of notifiable diseases. In the past, special surveillance systems for Hib were needed.[22] Varicella is a notifiable disease in some states, and those data are shared on an annual basis with the CDC.

The case definitions listed in the appendix to this chapter can serve as a guide to the clinician for reporting cases. However, for most of our vaccine-preventable diseases, cases should be reported to local and state health departments when suspected clinically so that interventions such as special outbreak control programs can be implemented rapidly. For example, a physician should not wait 14 days to evaluate whether a person with an illness clinically compatible with pertussis has a cough duration of 2 or more weeks. A suspected case should be reported immediately so that health authorities can help obtain and process appropriate laboratory specimens and appropriate control measures can be undertaken.

Delayed reporting can hamper measles control activities. Figure 7-1 shows the theoretical evolution of a measles outbreak.[23] At the time the first case can be diagnosed clinically (i.e., rash is manifest), the patient has already been communicable for two to four days during the prodrome. Thus, there may already be well persons who are incubating measles. If the clinician waits for testing of acute and convalescent phase sera to confirm the diagnosis, a process that can take as many as four weeks, the persons who are currently incubating measles will have become ill and exposed a third generation. Assuming an average interval between exposure to rash onset of 14 days, this third generation may become ill and have transmitted infection to a fourth generation by the time the serologic results for the first case become available.[24] Waiting for laboratory confirmation jeopardizes outbreak control because large numbers of persons are now exposed and at risk for measles. Therefore, it is better to err on the side of reporting a suspected case rather than await definitive confirmation before notifying health authorities.

In practice, reporting needs to be rapid if such reports lead to quick actions. For measles or polio, reporting should be immediate, as soon as a case is suspected. Because there is currently no vaccine for varicella and no major control program, however, varicella can generally be reported after the clinician believes the case is confirmed.

Active versus Passive Surveillance

Active surveillance involves the periodic solicitation of case reports from reporting sources such as physicians. In practice, this usually involves

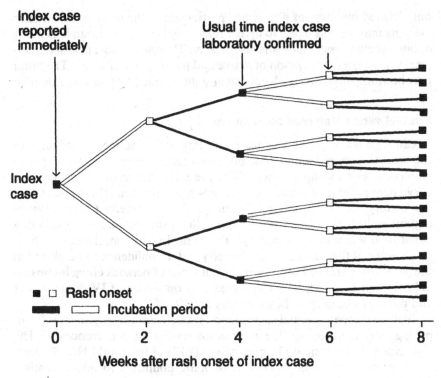

FIGURE 7-1.   Potential propagation of an outbreak. (From *J Am Coll Health* 1984; 33:64. Reprinted with permission.)

phone calls to providers designated by the state or local health department. These providers are usually chosen because they are likely to see cases of vaccine-preventable diseases and are willing to cooperate. In contrast, passive surveillance relies on health care providers to report on their own initiative. An evaluation of active and passive surveillance systems in Vermont and in Pierce County, Washington, indicated that physicians participating in the active system reported about twice the number of notifiable diseases per patient seen as physicians in the passive system.[25, 26] In a controlled evaluation of surveillance strategies in Monroe County, New York, active surveillance improved case reporting substantially. Telephone solicitation of cases increased reports of private physicians 4.6-fold over passive reporting, while mailout solicitation increased reports 2.6-fold.[27]

Despite the advantages of active surveillance, it is more expensive than passive surveillance. Active surveillance covers smaller populations since only limited numbers of physicians participate in the system. Thus, such systems may be less likely to detect relatively rare diseases such as many of our vaccine-preventable diseases today. Therefore, most health departments rely on a combination of active and passive surveillance. The latter may be stimulated through feedback in state newsletters and via the media.

Sentinel versus Universal Surveillance

Because of the expense of conducting large-scale active surveillance of the total U.S. population, some programs target sentinel sites for special emphasis. For example, since 1982, the CDC has conducted intensive surveillance and investigations of hepatitis in four sentinel counties (Denver County, Colorado; Jefferson County, Alabama; Pierce County, Washington; and Pinellas County, Florida).[26] Such surveillance suggested that hepatitis B was underreported by 50 percent. In addition, the comprehensive nature of the surveillance allowed greater confidence to be placed in the data which showed decreasing prominence of persons citing homosexual behavior as a risk factor and greater prominence of IV drug abusers and persons engaging in heterosexual activity.[28]

Well-developed sentinel surveillance systems are used by several European governments to provide information on disease occurrence.[10, 11] The Expanded Programme on Immunization (EPI) of the World Health Organization has encouraged many developing countries to adopt sentinel systems in which reports are accepted from selected providers within a community, generally the large hospitals.[29, 31] Such sentinel systems, while generally inexpensive may give biased information, depending upon how representative the sites are of the general community. For example, hospital-based systems are more likely to report sicker children who tend to be younger and unvaccinated than cases occurring in the community at large. Nevertheless, even these surveillance data are useful for evaluating trends and estimating the impact of the vaccination program.

Registries

Most disease-based surveillance in the United States relies on reports of disease from physicians to the CDC via local and state health departments. However, special registries are maintained for some diseases, which allow direct reporting of disease either to the CDC or to contractors. Until recently, the CDC maintained a registry that contained data on women vaccinated with rubella vaccines within 3 months of conception.[32] The women were followed prospectively to determine whether vaccination was associated with adverse pregnancy outcomes. In 1989, the registry was discontinued when adequate data had been accumulated to indicate that the risk of CRS following vaccination, if any, was less than 1.2 percent. A similar registry has been maintained to follow trends in reporting of subacute sclerosing panencephalitis (SSPE) to determine both whether vaccination against measles prevented SSPE and whether SSPE could be caused by vaccination.[33, 34] Data thus far show that SSPE has virtually disappeared from the United States.[35]

PHASES OF SURVEILLANCE

Immunization programs go through a series of phases from preprogram planning, to early implementation, to more extensive implementation, and finally to elimination or eradication. To assure the correct decisions are made, the information system needed will have to be tailored to each phase. At all times both surveillance and special studies are needed. However, the sophistication required of both types of information generally increases with each step.

Preprogram Planning

Prior to vaccine licensure, decisions must be made concerning how widely a vaccine may be used and which target populations should receive it. Surveillance data are important in providing information about age groups and special populations at risk, as well as information on complications that become important in evaluating cost/benefit. At this stage, data needs are usually quite simple, involving primarily information on age distribution and occurrence. For example, surveillance data were useful in designing strategies for vaccination against measles and rubella. Measles was a disease that affected many young children prior to school entry, while rubella was uncommon before school age (see Figure 7-2a).[4, 36, 37] Thus,

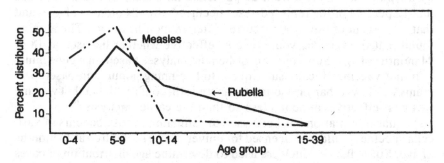

FIGURE 7-2a.   Age distributions of measles and rubella in the prevaccine era. (Measles 1960–1964, *Measles Surveillance Report* 11; rubella 1963–1967, *ADJC* 1969; 118:107.)

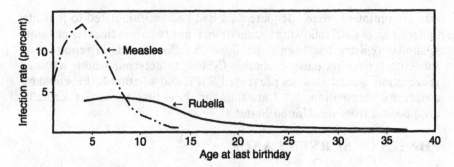

FIGURE 7-2b.   Estimated age specific infection rate of measles and rubella. (From *AJDC* 1969; 118:107. Reprinted with permission.)

immunization programs needed to target both children at 1 year of age as well as those in elementary school for measles. In contrast, vaccination efforts against rubella could be more focused toward school-age children, a population that is substantially easier to reach than preschool populations. In the case of measles and rubella, surveillance data were supplemented by special population-based studies that corroborated the validity of the surveillance information (see Figure 7-2b).[4, 36] Thus, although only a small proportion of cases were actually reported, the data were useful, along with data from special studies, in designing disease control strategies.

Surveillance data played an important role in the decision to license *Haemophilus b* polysaccharide vaccine (HbPV), which was based, in large part, on a cost-effectiveness analysis by Cochi et al.[38] The age breakdown for meningitis cases used in the analysis came from the CDC bacterial meningitis surveillance system. This system consisted of voluntary reports by hospital laboratories from 27 participating states. The data revealed that 19 percent of the reported cases occurred after 24 months of age, and that 29 percent of the cases occurred after 18 months of age. The authors found that the vaccine would be cost effective whether licensed at 18 or 24 months of age. Subsequent cost-benefit analyses based on a determination that vaccine efficacy subsequent to beginning population-based programs was lower than previously measured still confirmed that that vaccine was cost effective, although less so than the earlier analysis.[39]

Similar information has been used to estimate the cost/benefits of varicella vaccine should it be licensed for universal use in children at 15 months of age. Surveillance data were used to determine age distribution of cases and numbers and age distribution of varicella complications including encephalitis, Reye's syndrome, and death.[40, 41] Under the assumptions of the model which included 90 percent vaccine efficacy and 90 percent vaccine coverage, varicella vaccine would result in benefits of $6.9 saved for every $1 spent.[42]

Program Implementation

Once vaccines are licensed, there are a variety of information needs related to monitoring program impact and detecting program problems. These needs include data on: (1) the proportions of the target populations vaccinated and the characteristics of populations who have not been vaccinated; (2) changes in disease incidence and characteristics of remaining cases; and (3) the occurrence of adverse events following vaccination.

Vaccination Coverage

In the United States, vaccination is monitored through (1) direct measurement of immunization levels, (2) net distribution of doses as reported by manufacturers of specific vaccines, and (3) doses of vaccine administered in public-sector clinics.[1, 43, 44] Since 1978, national immunization levels have been assessed at school entry, kindergarten, or first grade. Each state health department reports the results of its assessment to the CDC, where a national estimate is calculated. School-enterer levels are not measured by sample survey but represent a census of the immunization status of *all* enterers. Each school must review the immunization status of each new enterer due to laws requiring specified immunizations prior to admission to school. Data from each school are usually compiled by school nurses or other school officials from immunization records on file for each student. State immunization program personnel perform sample validation surveys to confirm the school reports. Immunization levels for measles, mumps, rubella, polio, and DTP are shown in Table 7-2. Since the 1980–1981 school year, levels for measles, rubella, polio, and DTP have been 95 percent or greater. Similar results have been achieved for mumps, starting with the 1981–1982 school year.

The major advantage of this approach is that coverage levels are based on records rather than parental recall. Since many parents do not have immunization records of their children at home, persons doing telephone surveys or even home visits would have to list persons without records as unknown or rely on parental recall. Another advantage of the school-enterer assessment is that, because it is a census, there is no potential bias from sampling.

The major disadvantage is that immunization levels are measured several years after the vaccination should have been administered. For example, children at the time of school entry should have received 13 to 15

TABLE 7-2   Percent Immunized by Antigen: Kindergarten/1st Grade Immunization Status, 1980–1990, United States

Year	Measles	Mumps	Rubella	Polio	DTP/DT
1980/81	96	92	96	95	96
1981/82	97	95	97	96	96
1982/83	97	96	97	97	96
1983/84	98	97	98	97	97
1984/85	98	97	98	97	97
1985/86	97	96	97	96	96
1986/87	97	97	97	97	97
1987/88	98	98	98	97	97
1988/89	98	98	98	97	97
1989/90	98	98	98	97	97
1990/91[1]	98	98	98	97	97

[1] Provisional data as of 4/22/91

injections or oral administrations of vaccines. Of these, 11 to 12 are recommended for children 18 months of age or below.[45–48] A second problem relates to the validity of the records. Most states require physician confirmation of immunization status. However, if physicians rely on parental recall rather than records to certify immunization, falsely high immunization levels may be reported. Finally, because *haemophilus* vaccines are not required for school enterers, school-enterer levels cannot be used to assess coverage with this antigen.

Because of the desirability of information concerning immunization levels among preschool children, the United States has tried a variety of approaches, none of which are entirely satisfactory. From 1959 to 1985, the CDC contracted with the Bureau of the Census for an annual survey of households to determine immunization levels for all key age groups (United States Immunization Survey [USIS]).[43, 49] Beginning in 1972, the data were collected principally by telephone interview. Most of the answers were based on parental recall and the results were generally substantially lower than the results of the school-enterer assessments. In 1979, a question on whether parents were reading from records was added. Immunization levels based upon the approximately one-third of respondents with records more closely approximated results from the school enterer assessments.[43] Due to the cost, and concerns with the accuracy of the USIS, it was abandoned after 1985.

Other approaches to measuring preschool levels have included a statewide follow-up of a sample of children at two years of age who were selected from state birth certificates.[50] This technique also was abandoned

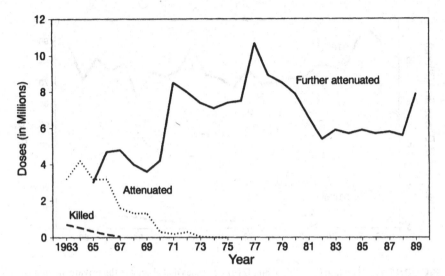

FIGURE 7-3.   Doses of measles virus vaccine distributed by year and vaccine type, United States, 1963–1989.

because response rates were frequently low, often less than 50 percent, casting concerns on the validity of the results.

Recently, a number of states have begun measuring immunization levels retrospectively using data obtained at school entry. Using date-specific information, immunization personnel calculate immunization levels for these enterers as of the date of their second birthday.[43, 44] While helpful in evaluating preschool immunization levels in the past and in monitoring trends, the method is not useful in estimating immunization coverage of current preschoolers.

Biologics Surveillance

Since 1962, the CDC has received data from vaccine manufacturers concerning the number of doses of vaccines they distributed minus the number of doses returned.[43, 51] Data on biologics distribution have been helpful in tracking the use of various types of measles vaccines (see Figure 7-3). In 1963, both killed and live attenuated (Edmonston B) vaccines were licensed. In 1965, further attenuated strains became available. By 1968, distribution of killed vaccine had ceased and by 1975 only further attenuated strains were being distributed. These data were used to recommend revaccination of persons that were vaccinated prior to 1968 with a vaccine of unknown type, since it might have been killed vaccine.[52] Biologics data

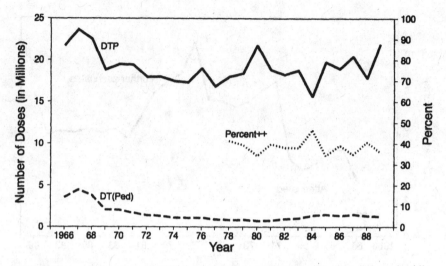

FIGURE 7-4.   Net number of DTP and DT (Ped) doses distributed in the private and public sectors and percent DTP administered in the public sector, United States 1966–1989. (From *Biologic Surveillance*, CDC.) Note: DTP vaccine administered data not reported to the CDC prior to 1978.

have also been useful in tracking DTP and DT use following adverse publicity about DTP beginning in 1982, which triggered concerns that vaccine coverage against pertussis would drop. Figure 7-4 shows that except for 1984—when there was a DTP shortage primarily due to the permanent departure from the market of one of the three DTP manufacturers and the temporary departure of another—DTP net distribution has remained relatively constant, while DT distribution has increased only slightly. The advantage of the biologics surveillance system is that data become available rapidly. If school-entry data were required, it would have taken about five years to obtain any information on infants born and immunized following the onset of the adverse publicity.

Public-sector Doses Administered

Since 1964, the CDC has received information on the number of doses administered by public-sector providers by age group.[43] Since 1987, data on dose in series (e.g., number of first doses of DTP administered, second doses of DTP administered, etc.) have also been forwarded to the CDC. The major uses of these data have been in monitoring the proportion of the population served by the public sector and in calculating rates of adverse events reported following vaccination in the public sector.

In 1982, the cost of DTP was about $0.15 in the public sector and about $0.37 in the private sector. By 1989, the prices had increased to $7.96 and $10.65, respectively. Providers cannot charge for vaccines purchased with federal funds. They must be provided free, although a nominal administration fee is allowable. The high prices of vaccines for parents having their children vaccinated by private physicians have raised concerns that such parents will seek immunization in public clinics, causing fragmentation of care and further straining limited public resources. Figure 7-4 shows the proportion of net doses of DTP distributed that were administered in the public sector. Although there have been anecdotal reports of such shifts, the national data through 1989 fail to reveal any discrete change from the routine pattern.

DISEASE SURVEILLANCE

The ultimate purpose of immunization is to prevent disease and complications of disease. Surveillance data on reported cases are critical to determine whether the program is having an impact, to assess why disease is still occurring, to evaluate whether new strategies are necessary, and to detect problem areas and populations that require more intensive program input.

As noted, disease surveillance systems initially need to be simple. Physician diagnosis is usually the case definition, and reported information may include date of onset or report, age, and state (and sometimes county) of residence. Such limited data have been useful in demonstrating the marked impact of vaccination on disease incidence, and for analyzing how best to reduce remaining morbidity. For example, surveillance data were used to develop policies to enhance rubella vaccination of postpubertal populations. Prior to vaccine licensure, persons 15 years of age or older accounted for less than 25 percent of reported cases (see Figure 7-5).[53] By the mid-1970s, incidence rates had declined among all age groups. However, persons in the childbearing age group accounted for the majority of cases. Further, there had not been discernible impact on reporting of CRS. By modifying the strategy to include susceptible postpubertal populations as well as children, the incidence of rubella and CRS declined to the extent that they are now on the verge of elimination.[5]

Surveillance data were instrumental in the spread of regulations to require vaccination for school children. School laws represented a linking of the vast resources of the educational establishment, with its access to almost all children, and a public health program with somewhat limited resources, but with the data to show that transmission of diseases

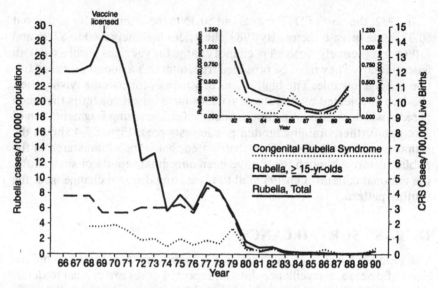

FIGURE 7-5. Incidence rates of reported rubella and congenital rubella syndrome (CRS) cases (reported to NCRSR) United States, 1966–1990 (provisional data, 1990).

such as measles in school settings represented a significant threat to those children. Beginning in the mid-1970s, surveillance data clearly showed that states without laws requiring vaccination at school entry had 1.7- to 2.0-fold higher incidence rates of reported measles than states with laws.[54] This information was extremely useful in the universal adoption of school-enterer requirements by showing legislators that laws could lead to significant impact. By the late 1970s, the epidemiology of measles had changed. Cases were more prominent in junior high school and high school students.[37] These students were not covered by recently enacted school-enterer laws since they were already enrolled when such regulations went into effect. This led to the adoption of comprehensive laws covering all students, from kindergarten through grade 12. Surveillance data showed such states had lower incidence rates for measles than other states, which led to the adoption of comprehensive laws by most states.[55, 56]

A critical aspect of the success of the school laws was the requirement that students not in compliance be excluded from school until they were immunized. It was often difficult to convince educators of the importance of exclusion. Surveillance data proved very useful by documenting that the measles incidence in states strictly enforcing laws with exclusion was substantially lower than measles incidence in other states.[56]

Recently, an analysis of reported mumps cases by age and by state demonstrated that marked increases in incidence were due to failure to vaccinate large numbers of older children and adolescents rather than to vaccine failure.[57] The highest incidence rates were in states without comprehensive school laws requiring mumps immunization. If vaccine failure were the predominant concern, increased incidence should have occurred in all states. Thus, evaluation of the role of vaccine failure was made without any data on vaccination status of cases.

Reports of increased numbers of cases can lead to special investigations. For example, the report of an outbreak of measles in Texarkana from 1970 to 1971 led to conclusive evidence that measles incidence in Arkansas students who were involved in a major measles control program was substantially lower than the incidence among students from Texas who were not covered by such a program.[58] This investigation helped spur greater control efforts in Texas. Similar investigations initiated through reports of unusual numbers of cases helped document that vaccination against measles at 12 months of age was not as effective as vaccination after 15 months of age.[59] Reports of outbreaks in vaccinated populations frequently lead to special investigations of vaccine efficacy.[19]

As programs mature and cases become more uncommon, surveillance tends to move from the simple passive collection of limited data on cases to more sophisticated individual case investigations by health department personnel. During these investigations, staff generally collect relevant clinical and laboratory data as well as information on disease complications, hospitalizations, and vaccination status, and other desired information such as potential sources and contacts of the case. Health department personnel may assist in collecting critical laboratory specimens such as acute and convalescent phase sera or providing transport media for bacterial and/or viral cultures. Special case investigation forms have been developed for congenital rubella syndrome, diphtheria, tetanus, pertussis, and hepatitis B, to name a few of the traditional vaccine-preventable diseases. Detailed information is collected on individual measles and polio cases. These data are used to analyze cases in greater depth, particularly with regard to health impact and problems with vaccination.

A major question in the control of vaccine-preventable diseases is whether a given case represents a failure of implementation of the vaccine strategy (a preventable case), or failure of the strategy (a nonpreventable case). For example, a preventable case of measles is disease in someone who was eligible for vaccine but was unvaccinated.

In the past, such persons must have been born after 1956, be at least 16 months of age, be a U.S. citizen, have no medical contraindications against measles vaccination, have no religious or philosophical exemptions to vaccination under state law, and have no evidence of measles immunity.[16] Measles immunity was defined as documented evidence of prior physician-diagnosed disease, receipt of live vaccine on or after the first birthday, or laboratory evidence of immunity. Analyses of cases by preventability status played a major role in new policy recommendations for more aggressive revaccination efforts. In recent years only a minority of cases were preventable and, especially among school-age children, vaccine failure was the predominant reason for nonpreventability.[60] Analyses of large school-age outbreaks in 1985 and 1986 ($\geq$100 cases) reported through the measles surveillance system demonstrated that as many as 69 percent of cases in such outbreaks were appropriately vaccinated. Of the school-age cases in these outbreaks, the age group in which the predominant transmission was occurring, a median of 71 percent were vaccinated, ranging up to 90 percent. These case reports, many of them initiated by physicians, played a crucial role in the recent recommendations for a routine two-dose schedule for measles and for more aggressive outbreak revaccination efforts.[47, 48]

ADVERSE EVENTS

Vaccination programs have an obligation to evaluate the safety as well as the efficacy of vaccines. Recommendations for the use of vaccines represent a balancing of benefits and risks. For example, information from surveillance of complications from vaccination against smallpox disease, coupled with information from surveillance of the disease, led to the recommendation to cease routine vaccination in 1971.[61, 62] The risks were believed to outweigh the benefits. The last case of smallpox was reported in the United States in 1949, and the disease was well on the way to eradication worldwide. In the absence of a risk from disease, there were real risks from vaccines. Reported rates of generalized vaccinia, eczema vaccinatum, and encephalitis were as high as 241.5, 39, and 12.3 per million primary doses, respectively.[63, 64]

Common adverse reactions caused by vaccine can usually be detected in prelicensure randomized, double-blind, placebo-controlled trials. However, the relationship of a rare event to the receipt of vaccine usually needs to be evaluated through postlicensure surveillance.[2] Such rare events usually are called adverse events temporally related to vaccine rather than adverse reactions, since the word reaction implies that it was caused by the vaccine. Often the rare events are not clinically distinguishable from events that occur in the absence of receipt of vaccine.

There is now a single system for monitoring adverse events following vaccination in the United States, the Vaccine Adverse Event Reporting

System (VAERS). Forms are available in the Food and Drug Administration's FDA Drug Bulletin and the *Physicians' Desk Reference,* or they may be obtained by calling VAERS at 1-800-822-7967. The VAERS is designed primarily to take reports from vaccine providers but allows for reporting of consumers directly. Consumers are urged to collaborate with providers in completing the VAERS form to assure that information is medically accurate. VAERS is designed to accept reports of adverse events following all vaccines.

Since March 1988, the National Childhood Vaccine Injury Act has required that vaccine providers report certain conditions to the Department of Health and Human Services.[65] Table 7-3 describes those reporting requirements. While only certain events following selected vaccines are specified by law for reporting, it is desirable to report all significant events following any vaccine.

There is substantial confusion concerning what passive adverse events monitoring systems can or cannot do. Their most useful function is to identify hypotheses for more detailed investigation in special studies. For example, reports of a cluster of Guillain-Barré syndrome cases, particularly within 2 to 3 weeks following vaccination with the A/New Jersey influenza vaccine (swine flu), led to careful epidemiologic studies implicating this vaccine as a cause of the syndrome.[66] Studies of subsequent vaccines have failed to show such relationships.[67] Passive surveillance has also been useful in detecting clusters of abscesses associated with bacterial contamination of single vials of DTP, a cluster of sterile abscesses associated with one manufacturer's product, and a cluster of sudden infant death syndrome (SIDS) after DTP.[68-70] The latter led to refined studies, most of which have failed to show any relationship of DTP to SIDS.[71] Passive systems are also used to monitor trends in reporting and can be used to evaluate some hypotheses. For example, forms from a previous system coordinated by the CDC, the Monitoring System for Adverse Events Following Immunization (MSAEFI), requested information on personal and family histories of seizures. Thus, MSAEFI data were used to determine that persons with such histories were significantly more likely to have seizures following DTP than persons without such histories.[72] Other hypotheses are currently being evaluated with information obtained from VAERS forms.

Despite the benefits of passive systems, they may not fulfill two important needs: (1) to measure accurately the incidence of adverse events, and (2) to determine whether a given event temporally related to a vaccine is caused by that vaccine. With passive reporting, there will almost always be underreporting of events. The legal requirements of the National Childhood Vaccine Injury Act should help stimulate reporting but it is still likely

TABLE 7-3   Events Following Immunization Required To Be Reported by the National Childhood Vaccine Injury Act

Vaccine	Event	Interval from Vaccination
DTP; P; DTP/Polio Combined	A. Anaphylaxis or anaphylactic shock	24 hours
	B. Encephalopathy (or encephalitis)[1]	7 days
	C. Shock-collapse or hypotonic-hyporesponsive collapse[1]	7 days
	D. Residual seizure disorder[1]	(See Aids to Interpretation[1])
	E. Any acute complication or sequela (including death) of above events	No limit
	F. Events in vaccines described in manufacturer's package insert as contraindications to additional doses of vaccine[2] (such as convulsions)	(See package insert)
Measles, Mumps, and Rubella; DT, Td, Tetanus Toxoid	A. Anaphylaxis or anaphylactic shock	24 hours
	B. Encephalopathy (or encephalitis)[1]	15 days for measles mumps, and rubella vaccines; 7 days for DT, Td and T toxoids
	C. Residual seizure disorder[1]	(See Aids to Interpretation[1])
	D. Any acute complication or sequela (including death) of above events.	No limit
	E. Events in vaccines described in manufacturer's package insert as contraindications to additional doses of vaccine[2]	(See package insert)
Oral Polio Vaccines	A. Paralytic poliomyelitis	
	• in a nonimmunodeficient recipient	30 days
	• in an immunodeficient recipient	6 months
	• in a vaccine-associated community case	No limit
	B. Any acute complication or sequela (including death) of above events	No limit
	C. Events in vaccines described in manufacturer's package insert as contraindications to additional doses of vaccine[2]	(See package insert)
Inactivated Polio Vaccine	A. Anaphylaxis or anaphylactic shock	24 hours
	B. Any acute complication or sequela (including death) of above event	No limit
	C. Events in vaccines described in manufacturer's package insert as contraindications to additional doses of vaccine[2]	(See package insert)

[1] AIDS TO INTERPRETATION: Shock-collapse or hypotonic-hyporesponsive collapse may be evidenced by signs or symptoms, such as decrease or loss of muscle tone, paralysis (partial or complete), hemiplegia, hemiparesis, loss of color or turning pale white or blue, unresponsiveness to environmental stimuli, depression of or loss of consciousness, prolonged sleeping with difficulty arousing, or cardiovascular or respiratory arrest.

Residual seizure disorder may be considered to have occurred if no other seizure or convulsion unaccompanied by fever or accompanied by a fever of less than 102°F occurred before the first seizure or convulsion after the administration of the vaccine involved.

and, if in the case of measles, mumps, or rubella containing vaccines, the first seizure or convulsion occurred within 15 days of vaccination *or*, in the case of any other vaccine, the first seizure or convulsion occurred within 3 days of vaccination,

and if two or more seizures or convulsions occurred within 1 year from vaccination which were afebrile or were accompanied by a fever of less than 102°F.

The terms seizure and convulsion include grand mal, petit mal, absence, myoclonic, tonic-clonic, and focal motor seizures and signs.

Encephalopathy means any significant acquired abnormality of, or injury to, or impairment of function of the brain. Among the frequent manifestations of encephalopathy are focal and diffuse neurological signs, increased intracranial pressure, or changes lasting at least 6 hours in level of consciousness, with or without convulsions. The neurologic signs and symptoms of encephalopathy may be temporary with complete recovery, or may result in various degrees of permanent impairment. Signs and symptoms such as high-pitched and unusual screaming, persistent inconsolable crying, and bulging fontanel are compatible with an encephalopathy, but in and of themselves are not conclusive evidence of encephalopathy. Encephalopathy usually can be documented by slow wave activity on an electroencephalogram.

[2] The health care provider who administered the vaccine must refer to the *contraindication* section of the manufacturer's package insert for each vaccine.

that reporting will not be complete. Even if reporting were complete, assessing causation may be difficult. This is because many adverse events do not have specific clinical or laboratory characteristics to differentiate them from events that occur in the absence of vaccination. To determine causation epidemiologically requires the demonstration that either vaccinees are more likely to suffer the event than nonvaccinees (cohort design), or that persons with the event are more likely to have a history of recent vaccination than persons without the event (case-control design). Passive systems do not have built-in control groups to allow measurement of the incidence of the event in the absence of vaccination. Therefore, true determination of causation usually requires special studies. Causation may be accepted in the absence of special studies if the event is clinically distinctive (e.g., vaccine-associated polio) or if organisms are cultured from normally sterile body sites (e.g., BCG-induced osteomyelitis).[73, 74]

The limitations of passive reporting systems have been described in detail.[75] Nevertheless, since they cover surveillance of large populations, they remain the only practical means of identifying rare adverse events.

ERADICATION/ELIMINATION

The eradication of disease—usually defined as the permanent absence of disease—or elimination of disease—usually defined as absence of disease but requiring constant vigilance because of the danger of repeated importations with reestablishment of indigenous transmission—requires more detailed information. Surveillance systems must be strengthened so that every case can be detected rapidly. Therefore, active surveillance plays a more prominent role than in routine surveillance settings. Individual case investigations are essential and laboratory confirmation becomes increasingly important.[76] Classifying cases as preventable or nonpreventable becomes a guide to further efforts.[60] Determining the reasons for nonpreventability is a critical part of the information needed for further strategy changes. Outbreak control is a crucial aspect of elimination/eradication efforts.[37] Thus, the surveillance system must detect cases rapidly. During outbreaks, surveillance systems are intensified to determine geographic zones for implementing control efforts and to select appropriate target populations for vaccination. Any eradication/elimination effort requires special coordination between physicians and health departments to assure success.

EVALUATION

The Centers for Disease Control has developed extensive guidelines for the evaluation of public health surveillance systems.[77, 78] Such evaluations consist of determining usefulness, simplicity, flexibility, acceptability, sensitivity in detecting the true number of cases or epidemics, predictive value positive of reported cases (i.e., the proportion of cases reported that are true cases), representativeness of reported cases, timeliness of reporting, and cost-effectiveness. With regard to immunization, major questions have revolved around sensitivity and predictive value positive. Attempts at determining sensitivity have been frustrated by not having good estimates of the total burden of disease during the program. As noted earlier, prior to beginning control, such estimates for diseases like measles have been available allowing sensitivity determination. However, once the disease burden decreases due to vaccination, the total remaining burden is difficult to estimate. Particular use has been made of the Chandrasekar and Deming method of estimating total incidence with regard to tetanus deaths and congenital rubella syndrome.[5, 79] This method requires two independent surveillance systems detecting the same illness, and measures the degree of overlap to estimate the total burden. It is similar to capture-recapture systems used to estimate animal populations. Efficiency of adverse events reporting can be evaluated if population-based estimates based on prior studies are available. Predictive value positive studies have used gold standards such as laboratory confirmation to evaluate the proportion of cases, given a particular case definition, that are laboratory-confirmed.[18]

CONCLUSIONS

Success in immunization requires success in developing an adequate information base. While special studies are important, there is no substitute for surveillance systems. Such systems help to evaluate health impact, monitor trends in reported disease and adverse events, and identify areas for more intense investigation. Surveillance data alone have played major roles in immunization strategy changes. Successful surveillance relies on cooperation by health care providers and health departments. While filling out forms and reporting cases may be viewed as a burden by some, such information in the aggregate becomes an important part of the knowledge base used to refocus implementation efforts and, potentially, to change strategies. Reporting by all physicians is particularly important when reported cases lead to aggressive control actions such as outbreak control. Rapid reporting even when cases are not confirmed can help health departments assure needed laboratory specimens are collected and allow control measures to be undertaken before disease spreads to the point where it is difficult to contain. In conclusion, any immunization program worth instituting is worth monitoring. Surveillance represents constant vigilance to assure effective control or elimination.

ACKNOWLEDGMENTS

The authors would like to acknowledge the contributions of Terence Chorba, who provided many reference materials; Edward Brink, Stephen Cochi, Donald Eddins, and Stephen Thacker, who provided helpful comments; Sonia Russell, who developed the graphics; and Virginia Lee, who typed the manuscript.

Notes

1. Eddins, D. L. 1987. *Immunization Status of the Nation's 2-year-old Children,* 63–66. Proceedings of the 21st Immunization Conference, New Orleans, Louisiana, June 8–11.
2. Stetler, H. C., J. R. Mullen, J. P. Brennon, J. R. Livengood, W. A. Orenstein, and A. R. Hinman. 1987. Monitoring system for adverse events following immunization. *Vaccine* 5:169–174.
3. Hinman, A. R. 1988. DTP vaccine litigation update. *Am J Dis Child* 142:1275.
4. Langmuir, A. D. 1962. Medical importance of measles. *Am J Dis Child* 103:54–56.
5. Cochi, S. L., L. E. Edmonds, K. Dyer et al. 1989. Congenital rubella syndrome in the United States, 1970–1985: on the verge of elimination. *Am J Epidemiol* 129:349–361.
6. Centers for Disease Control. 1987. Pertussis surveillance: United States, 1984 and 1985. *MMWR* 36:168–171.
7. Royal College of General Practitioners. 1981. Effect of a low pertussis vaccination uptake on a large community. *Br Med J* 282:23–26.
8. Grog, P. R., J. J. Crowder, and J. F. Robbins. 1981. Effect of vaccination on severity of dissemination of whooping cough. *Br Med J* 282:1925–1928.
9. Stewart, G. T. 1981. Whooping cough in relation to other childhood infections in 1977–79 in the United Kingdom. *J. Epidemiol Community Health* 35:139–145.
10. Thacker, S. B., and R. L. Berkelman. 1988. Public health surveillance in the United States. *Epidemiol Rev* 10:164–190.
11. Eylenbosch, W. J., and N. D. Noah, eds. 1988. *Surveillance in Health and Disease,* 1–286. Oxford: Oxford University Press.
12. Vogt, R. September 1988. Disease surveillance: Who reports? *Disease Control Bulletin,* Vermont Department of Health.
13. Sacks, J. J. 1985. Utilization of case definitions and laboratory reporting in the surveillance of notifiable communicable diseases in the United States. *Am J Public Health* 75:1420–1422.
14. Choi, K., and S. B. Thacker. 1981. An evaluation of influenza mortality

surveillance, 1962–1979. I. Time series forecasts of expected pneumonia and influenza deaths. *Am J Epidemiol* 113:215–226.
15. Brachman, P. S. Surveillance. In Evans, A. S. and H. H. Feldman, eds. 1982. *Bacterial Infections of Humans,* 49–61. New York: Plenum Medical.
16. Centers for Disease Control. 1982. Classification of measles cases and categorization of measles elimination programs. *MMWR* 31:707–711.
17. Centers for Disease Control. 1990. Case definitions for public health surveillance. *MMWR* 39(No. RR-13):[1–43].
18. Patriarca, P. A., R. J. Biellik, G. Sanders et al. 1988. Sensitivity and specificity of clinical case definitions for pertussis. *Am J Public Health* 78:833–836.
19. Orenstein, W. A., R. H. Bernier, and A. R. Hinman. 1988. Assessing vaccine efficacy in the field: further observations. *Epidemiol Rev* 10:212–241.
20. Chorba, T. L., R. L. Berkelman, S. K. Safford, N. P. Gibbs, and H. F. Hull. 1989. The reportable diseases. I. Mandatory reporting of infectious diseases by clinicians. *JAMA* 262:3018–3026.
21. Thacker, S. B., K. Choi, and P. S. Brachman. 1983. The surveillance of infectious diseases. *JAMA* 249:1181–1185.
22. Schlech, W. F., III. J. I. Ward, J. O. Band, A. Hightower, D. W. Fraser, and C. V. Broome. 1985. Bacterial meningitis in the United States, 1978 through 1981: the National Bacterial Meningitis Surveillance Study. *JAMA* 253:1949–1954.
23. Amler, R. W., and W. A. Orenstein. 1984. Measles: Current status and outbreak control on campus. *J Am Coll Health* 33:64–66.
24. Hope Simpson, R. E. 1952. Infectiousness of communicable diseases in the household (measles, chickenpox, and mumps). *Lancet* 1952. 2:549–554.
25. Vogt, R. L., D. LaRue, D. N. Klaucke, and D. A. Jillson. 1983. Comparison of an active and passive surveillance system of primary care providers for hepatitis, measles, rubella, and salmonellosis in Vermont. *Am J Public Health* 73:795–797.
26. Alter, M. J., A. Mares, S. C. Hadler, and J. E. Maynard. 1987. The effect of underreporting on the apparent incidence and epidemiology of acute viral hepatitis. *Am J Epidemiol* 125:133–139.
27. Thacker, S. B., S. Redmond, R. B. Rothenberg, S. B. Spitz, K. Choi, and M. C. White. 1986. A controlled trial of disease surveillance strategies. *Am J Prev Med* 2:345–350.
28. Centers for Disease Control. 1988. Changing patterns of groups at high risk for hepatitis B in the United States. *MMWR* 39:429–432, 437.
29. Expanded Programme on Immunization: measles surveillance methodology. *Wkly Epidem Rec* 1986; 25:191–193.
30. Dondero, T. 1984. EPI target disease surveillance and disease reduction targets. Expanded Programme on Immunization, EPI/GEN/84/6. Geneva, Switzerland: World Health Organization.
31. Expanded Programme on Immunization. 1986. Evaluation and monitoring of National immunization programmes. EPI/GEN/86/4 Rev. 1. Geneva, Switzerland: World Health Organization.

32. Centers for Disease Control. 1989. Rubella vaccination during pregnancy. United States, 1971–1988. *MMWR* 38:289–293.
33. Modlin, J. F., J. T. Jabbour, J. J. Witte, and N. A. Halsey. 1977. Epidemiologic studies of measles, measles vaccine, and subacute sclerosing panencephalitis. *Pediatr* 59:505–512.
34. Halsey, N. A., Modlin, J. F., and J. T. Jabbour. Subacute sclerosing panencephalitis: an epidemiologic review. In Stevens, J. G., G. J. Todoro, and C. F. Fox, eds. 1978. *Persistent Viruses*, 101–104. Proceedings of the ICN-UCLA Symposia on molecular and cellular biology, vol. XI. New York: Academic Press.
35. Bloch, A. B., W. A. Orenstein, H. C. Stetler et al. 1985. Health impact of measles vaccination in the United States. *Pediatr* 76:524–532.
36. Witte, J. J., A. W. Karchner, G. Case, R. L. Herrmann, E. Abrutyn, I. Kussanoff, and J. A. Neill. 1969. Epidemiology of rubella. *Am J Dis Child* 118:107–111.
37. Centers for Disease Control. September 1982. *Measles Surveillance Report No. 11, 1977–1981.* Atlanta, Ga.: CDC.
38. Cochi, S. L., C. V. Broome, and A. W. Hightower. 1985. Immunization of U.S. children with *Hemophilus influenzae* type b polysaccharide vaccine: A cost-effectiveness model of strategy assessment. *JAMA* 253:521–529.
39. Hay, J. W., and R. S. Daum. 1987. Cost-benefit analysis of two strategies for prevention of *Haemophilus influenzae* type b infection. *Pediatr* 80:319–329.
40. Preblud, S. R. 1981. Age-specific risks of varicella complications. *Pediatr* 68:14–17.
41. Preblud, S. R., W. A. Orenstein, and K. J. Bart. 1984. Varicella: clinical manifestations, epidemiology and health impact in children. *Ped Inf Dis* 3:505–509.
42. Preblud, S. R., W. A. Orenstein, J. P. Koplan, K. J. Bart, and A. R. Hinman. 1985. A benefit-cost analysis of a childhood varicella vaccination programme. *Postgrad Med J* 61(suppl. 4):17–22.
43. Eddins, D. L. 1982. *Indicators of Immunization Status*, 47–55. 17th Immunization Conference Proceedings, Atlanta, Georga, May 18–19.
44. Eddins, D. L. 1983. *Present Systems That Provide Indicators of Immunization Status of Preschool Children*, 83–84. 18th Immunization Conference Proceedings, Atlanta, Georgia, May 16–19.
45. Centers for Disease Control. 1989. Recommendations of the Immunization Practices Advisory Committee (ACIP): general recommendations on immunization. *MMWR* 38:205–214, 219–227.
46. Centers for Disease Control. *Haemophilus* b conjugate vaccines for prevention of *Haemophilus influenzae* type b disease among infants and children two months of age and older: recommendations of the Immunization Practices Advisory Committee (ACIP). *MMWR* 40 (no RR-1):[1–7].
47. Committee on Infectious Diseases, American Academy of Pediatrics. 1989. Measles: Reassessment of the current immunization policy. *Pediatrics* 84:1110–1113.

48. Centers for Disease Control. 1989. Recommendations of the Immunization Practices Advisory Committee (ACIP): measles prevention. *MMWR* 38 (No. S-9):[1–18].
49. Centers for Disease Control. 1959–1985. Published and unpublished data, U.S. Immunization Survey Reports, Division of Immunization.
50. Centers for Disease Control. 1972. Guidelines for assessing immunity levels, USDHEW, PHS, CDC, Immunization Branch. Atlanta.
51. Centers for Disease Control. 1987. Biologics Surveillance Report No. 93, January to December, Division of Immunization. Atlanta.
52. Centers for Disease Control. 1987. Recommendations of the Immunization Practices Advisory Committee (ACIP): measles prevention. *MMWR* 36:409–418, 423–425.
53. Orenstein, W. A., K. J. Bart, A. R. Hinman et al. 1984. The opportunity and obligation to eliminate rubella from the United States. *JAMA* 251:1988–1994.
54. Orenstein, W. A., N. A. Halsey, G. F. Hayden et al. 1978. Current status of measles in the United States, 1973–1977. *J Infect Dis* 137:847–853.
55. Centers for Disease Control. 1978. Measles and school immunization requirements: United States 1978. *MMWR* 27:303–304.
56. Robbins, R. B., A. D. Brandling Bennett, and A. R. Hinman. 1981. Low measles incidence: association with enforcement of school immunization laws. *Am J Public Health* 91:270–274.
57. Cochi, S. C., S. R. Preblud, and W. A. Orenstein. 1988. Perspectives on the relative resurgence of mumps in the United States. *Am J Dis Child* 142:499–507.
58. Landrigan, P. J. 1972. Epidemic measles in a divided city. *JAMA* 221:567–570.
59. Orenstein, W. A., L. Markowitz, S. R. Preblud, A. R. Hinman, A. Tomasi, and K. J. Bart. 1986. Appropriate age for measles vaccination in the United States. *Dev Biol Stand* 65:13–21.
60. Markowitz, L. E., S. R. Preblud, W. A. Orenstein, E. Z. Rovira, N. C. Adams, C. E. Hawkins, and A. R. Hinman. 1989. Patterns of transmission in measles outbreaks in the United States, 1985–1986. *NEJM* 320:75–81.
61. Centers for Disease Control. 1971. Public Health Service recommendation on smallpox vaccination. *MMWR* 20:339.
62. Centers for Disease Control. 1971. Vaccination against smallpox in the United States: a reevaluation of the risks and benefits. *MMWR* 20:339–345.
63. Lane, M. J., R. L. Ruben, J. M. Neff, and J. D. Millar. 1969. Complications of smallpox vaccination, 1968: national surveillance in the United States. *NEJM* 281:1201–1208.
64. Lane, J. M., R. L. Ruben, J. M. Neff, and J. D. Millar. 1970. Complications of smallpox vaccination, 1968: results of ten statewide surveys. *J Infect Dis* 122:303–309.
65. Centers for Disease Control. 1988. National Childhood Vaccine Injury Act: requirements for permanent vaccination records and for reporting of selected events after vaccination. *MMWR* 37:197–200.
66. Schonberger, L. B., D. J. Bregman, J. Z. Sullivan-Bolyai et al. 1979. Guillain-Barré syndrome following vaccination in the national influenza immunization program, United States 1976–1977. *Am J Epidemiol* 110:105–123.

67. Kaplan, J. E., P. Katona, E. S. Hurwitz, and L. B. Schonberger. 1982. Guillain-Barré syndrome in the United States, 1979–1980 and 1980–1981: lack of an association with influenza vaccination. *JAMA* 248:698–700.
68. Stetler, H. C., P. L. Garbe, D. M. Dwyer et al. 1985. Outbreaks of Group A streptococcal abscesses following diphtheria-tetanus toxoid-pertussis vaccination. *Pediatrics* 75:299–303.
69. Bernier, R. H., J. A. Frank, Jr., and T. F. Nolan, Jr. 1981. Abscesses complicating DTP vaccination. *Am J Dis Child* 135:826–828.
70. Bernier, R. H., J. A. Frank, Jr., T. J. Dondero, Jr., and P. Turner. 1982. Diphtheria-tetanus toxoids-pertussis vaccination and sudden infant deaths in Tennessee. *J Pediatr* 101:419–421.
71. Griffin, M. R., W. A. Ray, J. R. Livengood, and W. Schaffner. 1988. Risk of sudden infant death syndrome after immunization with the diphtheria-tetanus-pertussis vaccine. *NEJM* 319:618–623.
72. Stetler, H. C., W. A. Orenstein, K. J. Bart, E. W. Brink, J. P. Brennan, and A. R. Hinman. 1985. History of convulsions and use of pertussis vaccine. *J Pediatr* 107:175–179.
73. Nkowane, B. M., S. G. F. Wassilak, W. A. Orenstein, K. J. Bart, L. B. Schonberger, A. R. Hinman, and O. M. Kew. 1987. Vaccine-associated paralytic poliomyelitis: United States, 1973 through 1984. *JAMA* 257:1335–1340.
74. Rosenthal, S. R. 1980. *BCG Vaccine: Tuberculosis to Cancer*, 261–262. Littleton, Mass.: PSG Publishing Company, Inc.
75. Centers for Disease Control. February 1989. *Adverse Events Following Immunization*. Surveillance report no. 3, 1985–1986. Atlanta.
76. Hinman, A. R., C. D. Kirby, D. L. Eddins, W. A. Orenstein, R. H. Bernier, P. M. Turner, and K. J. Bart. 1983. Elimination of indigenous measles from the United States. *Rev Infect Dis* 5:538–545.
77. Centers for Disease Control. 1988. Guidelines for evaluating surveillance systems. *MMWR* 37 (S-5):[1–18].
78. Thacker, S. B., R. G. Parrish, and F. L. Trowbridge. 1988. Surveillance coordination group: A method for evaluating systems of epidemiological surveillance. *Wld Hlt Statist Quart* 41:11–18.
79. Sutter, R. W., S. L. Cochi, E. W. Brink, and B. I. Sirotkin. 1990. Assessment of vital statistics and surveillance data for monitoring tetanus mortality: United States, 1979–1984. *Am J Epidemiol* 131:132–142.

APPENDIX*

Diphtheria

Clinical Case Definition
An upper respiratory tract illness characterized by sore throat, low-grade fever, and an adherent membrane of the tonsil(s), pharynx, and/or nose without other apparent cause (as reported by a health professional).

Laboratory Criteria for Diagnosis
Isolation of *Corynebacterium diphtheriae* from a clinical specimen.

Case Classification
Probable: Meets the clinical case definition, is not laboratory confirmed, and is not epidemiologically linked to a laboratory-confirmed case.

Confirmed: Meets the clinical case definition and is either laboratory confirmed or epidemiologically linked to a laboratory-confirmed case.

Comment
Cutaneous diphtheria should not be reported.

Tetanus

Clinical Case Definition
Acute onset of hypertonia and/or painful muscular contractions (usually of the muscles of the jaw and neck) and generalized muscle spasms without other apparent medical cause (as reported by a health professional).

---

* Modified from Reference 17.

Case Classification
Confirmed: A case that meets the clinical case definition.

Pertussis

Clinical Case Definition
A cough illness lasting at least two weeks with one of the following: paroxysms of coughing, inspiratory "whoop," or post-tussive vomiting—and without other apparent cause (as reported by a health professional).

Laboratory Criteria for Diagnosis
Isolation of Bordetella pertussis from clinical specimen.

Case Classification
Probable: Meets the clinical case definition, is not laboratory confirmed, and is not epidemiologically linked to a laboratory-confirmed case.

Confirmed: A clinically compatible case that is laboratory confirmed or epidemiologically linked to a laboratory-confirmed case.

Comment
The clinical case definition above is appropriate for endemic or sporadic cases. In outbreak settings, a case may be defined as a cough illness lasting at least two weeks (as reported by a health professional). Because direct fluorescent antibody testing of nasopharyngeal secretions has been shown in some studies to have low sensitivity and variable specificity, it should not be relied on as a criterion for laboratory confirmation.

Poliomyelitis, Paralytic

Clinical Case Definition
Acute onset of a flaccid paralysis of one or more limbs with decreased or absent tendon reflexes in the affected limbs, without other apparent cause, and without sensory or cognitive loss (as reported by a physician).

Case Classification
Probable: A case that meets the clinical case definition.

Confirmed: A case that meets the clinical case definition and in which the patient has a neurologic deficit 60 days after onset of initial symptoms, has died, or has unknown follow-up status.

Comment
All suspected cases of paralytic poliomyelitis are reviewed by a panel of expert consultants before final classification occurs. Only confirmed cases are included in Table 1 in the *MMWR*. Suspected cases are enumerated in a footnote to the *MMWR* table.

Measles

Clinical Case Definition
An illness characterized by all of the following clinical features:

- A generalized rash lasting ≥ 3 days
- A temperature ≥ 38.3°C (101°F)
- Cough, or coryza, or conjunctivitis

Laboratory Criteria for Diagnosis
- Isolation of measles virus from a clinical specimen, or
- Significant rise in measles antibody level by any standard serologic assay, or
- Positive serologic test for measles IgM antibody

Case Classification
Suspect: Any rash illness with fever.

Probable: Meets the clinical case definition, has no or noncontributory serologic or virologic testing, and is not epidemiologically linked to a probable or confirmed case.

Confirmed: A case that is laboratory confirmed or that meets the clinical case definition and is epidemiologically linked to a confirmed or probable case. A laboratory-confirmed case does not need to meet the clinical case definition.

Comment
Two probable cases that are epidemiologically linked would be considered confirmed, even in the absence of laboratory confirmation.

Mumps

Clinical Case Definition
An illness with acute onset of unilateral or bilateral tender, self-limited swelling of the parotid or other salivary gland, lasting ≥ 2 days, and without other apparent cause (as reported by a health professional).

Laboratory Criteria for Diagnosis
- Isolation of mumps virus from clinical specimen, or
- Significant rise in mumps antibody level by any standard serologic assay, or
- Positive serologic test for mumps IgM antibody

Case Classification

Probable: Meets the clinical case definition, has no or noncontributory serologic or virologic testing, and is not epidemiologically linked to a confirmed or probable case.

Confirmed: A case that is laboratory confirmed or that meets the clinical case definition and is epidemiologically linked to a confirmed or probable case. A laboratory-confirmed case does not need to meet the clinical case definition.

Comment

Two probable cases that are epidemiologically linked would be considered confirmed, even in the absence of laboratory confirmation.

Rubella

Clinical Case Definition

An illness with all of the following characteristics:

- Acute onset of generalized maculopapular rash
- Temperature >37.2°C (>99°F), if measured
- Arthralgia/arthritis, or lymphadenopathy, or conjunctivitis

Cases meeting the measles case definition are excluded. Also excluded are cases with serology compatible with recent measles virus infection.

Laboratory Criteria for Diagnosis
- Isolation of rubella virus, or
- Significant rise in rubella antibody level by any standard serologic assay, or
- Positive serologic test for rubella IgM antibody

Case Classification

Suspect: Any generalized rash illness of acute onset.

Probable: A case that meets the clinical case definition, has no or noncontributory serologic or virologic testing, and is not epidemiologically linked to a laboratory-confirmed case.

Confirmed: A case that is laboratory confirmed or that meets the clinical case definition and is epidemiologically linked to a laboratory-confirmed case.

Rubella Syndrome, Congenital

Clinical Description

An illness of newborns resulting from rubella infection in utero and characterized by symptoms from the following categories:

(A) Cataracts/congenital glaucoma, congenital heart disease, loss of hearing, pigmentary retinopathy.

Associated symptoms may be:

(B) Purpura, splenomegaly, jaundice, microcephaly, mental retardation, meningoencephalitis, radiolucent bone disease.

Clinical Case Definition
Presence of any defects or laboratory data consistent with congenital rubella infection (as reported by a health professional).

Laboratory Criteria for Diagnosis
- Isolation of rubella virus, or
- Demonstration of rubella-specific IgM antibody, or
- An infant's rubella antibody level that persists above and beyond that expected from passive transfer of maternal antibody (i.e., rubella HI titer that does not drop at the expected rate of a twofold dilution per month)

Case Classification
Possible: A case with some compatible clinical findings but not meeting the criteria for a compatible case.

Compatible: A case that is not laboratory confirmed and that has any two complications listed in (A) above, or one complication from (A) and one from (B).

Confirmed: A clinically compatible case that is laboratory confirmed.

Comment
In compatible cases, either or both of the eye-related findings (cataracts and congenital glaucoma) count as a single complication.

Haemophilus Influenzae (Invasive Disease)

Clinical Description
Invasive disease due to *Haemophilus influenzae* may produce any of several clinical syndromes, including meningitis, bacteremia, epiglottitis, or pneumonia.

Laboratory Criterion for Diagnosis
- Isolation of *H. influenzae* from a normally sterile site.

Case Classification
Probable: A clinically compatible illness with detection of *H. influenzae* type b antigen in cerebrospinal fluid.

Confirmed: A clinically compatible illness that is culture confirmed.

Comment
Antigen test results in urine or serum are unreliable for diagnosis of *H. influenzae* disease.

Hepatitis B

Clinical Case Definition
An illness with a) discrete onset of symptoms and b) jaundice or elevated serum aminotransferase levels.

Laboratory Criterion for Diagnosis
- Hepatitis B: IgM anti-HBc-positive (if done) or HBsAg-positive, and IgM anti-HAV-negative (if done).

Case Classification
Confirmed: A case that meets the clinical case definition and is laboratory confirmed.

Comment
Chronic carriage or chronic hepatitis should not be reported.

8

Surveillance of Acquired Immunodeficiency Syndrome (AIDS)

Ruth L. Berkelman, James W. Buehler,
and Timothy J. Dondero, Jr.

Surveillance for acquired immunodeficiency syndrome (AIDS) has been one of the most dynamic surveillance systems in the history of public health. Since its inception in 1981, the system has had to adapt to enormous changes, including (1) a rapid increase in knowledge, such as the discovery of the etiologic agent for AIDS, human immunodeficiency virus (HIV), in 1983, and the recognition of a wide and expanding spectrum of diseases associated with HIV infection; (2) the introduction of a diagnostic test for HIV infection in 1985; and (3) changes and variations in diagnostic and treatment practices for the array of cancers and opportunistic infections associated with HIV. In addition, the progressive rise in the number of cases has strained the ability of both health care providers and health departments to assure complete reporting of cases and to manage the expanding database. Issues surrounding social stigmatization and discrimination have also required extraordinary measures to safeguard the identity of reported individuals.

Since the discovery of AIDS, reporting of cases has been integral to surveillance of the HIV/AIDS epidemic. However, as more has been learned about the disease, including its long latency period (median approximately 10 years), other surveillance systems have been developed to supplement AIDS case reporting. A larger role for medical care records (e.g., hospital discharge data, Medicaid records) and vital statistics has been developed to assess the burden of HIV-related disease. The "family" of seroprevalence surveys, a group of surveys and studies of HIV infection in selected sentinel populations and special settings throughout the United States, was initiated in 1987 to provide more accurate information on HIV incidence and prevalence trends. HIV reporting of individuals is currently

108

being used by some states to provide detailed data on HIV-infected individuals as well as to provide a framework for a variety of prevention and health care measures. In several areas, special surveillance methods are being developed to monitor the full spectrum of illness occurring in persons with HIV infection, filling the gap between surveillance for HIV infection and AIDS cases. Surveillance for HIV/AIDS continues to evolve rapidly, as knowledge of HIV disease is advanced and surveillance techniques are refined.

AIDS CASE SURVEILLANCE

Background

In June 1981, the first cases of *Pneumocystis carinii* pneumonia (PCP) were recognized in five homosexual men in Los Angeles, and the Centers for Disease Control (CDC) began surveillance for the constellation of diseases, including PCP, Kaposi's sarcoma, and other opportunistic diseases, associated with acquired immunodeficiency syndrome (AIDS). The CDC developed a surveillance case definition for this syndrome and initially received case reports directly from both health care providers and state and local health departments. As the epidemic became more widespread, state and local health departments assumed increased responsibility for AIDS surveillance, with the Council of State and Territorial Epidemiologists (CSTE) making AIDS a nationally notifiable condition in 1983. By 1984, almost all states had laws or regulations requiring physicians and other health care providers to report AIDS cases directly to state or local health departments, and these health departments then shared those reports with the CDC. Thus, the surveillance system was initiated as it had been for other newly recognized diseases, including toxic shock syndrome and legionnaires' disease, evolving from a quickly implemented, ad hoc reporting system to a formal, national network involving extensive collaboration between the CDC and state and territorial health departments. However, unlike these other "new" diseases, which were comparatively rare causes of death, over 115,000 cumulative cases had been reported to the CDC before the end of the decade, including 66,000 deaths.

The goals of AIDS surveillance have been to monitor trends in severe morbidity and mortality due to infection with HIV, to assess the need for health care services, and to guide the public health response to the HIV/AIDS epidemic. Early in the epidemic, AIDS surveillance identified cases for epidemiologic research; a case-control study using cases identified through AIDS surveillance determined the principal modes of transmission and directly led to knowledge of effective prevention measures before the etiology of the disease was discovered.[1] AIDS surveillance has also provided the basis for projecting the future course of the HIV/AIDS epidemic and, through mathematical modeling, has helped to estimate the total prevalence of HIV infection.[2]

Case Definition

Well before the etiologic agent for AIDS was identified, AIDS was defined by a group of conditions (e.g., PCP, Kaposi's sarcoma) that was at least moderately indicative of a defect in cell-mediated immunity and that occurred in persons with no other known causes for diminished resistance to the condition.[3] When HIV was identified as the causative agent for AIDS and laboratory tests to detect the HIV antibody became available, the case definition was expanded to include additional "indicator" conditions in persons with laboratory evidence for HIV infection. In 1985, disseminated histoplasmosis, chronic isoporiasis, and certain non-Hodgkins lymphomas in HIV-infected persons were added to the case definition.[4] In 1987, based on greater knowledge of the clinical presentations of AIDS, the definition was expanded again to include HIV-infected persons with extrapulmonary tuberculosis, HIV encephalopathy, and HIV wasting syndrome.[5] In addition, the 1987 revision of the case definition allowed for presumptive as well as definitive diagnosis of certain indicator diseases in HIV-infected individuals to accommodate changing diagnostic practices.

Subsequent to the 1987 case definition revision, almost 30 percent of the cases have met only the additional criteria of the revision (see Fig. 8-1). The expansion of the definition in 1987 led to a greater increase in the number of reported cases among blacks and Hispanics, women, and intravenous drug users compared with other groups resulting in similar proportions of HIV-infected persons with severe immunodeficiency.[6] In particular, the abrupt increase in reported cases associated with the revision has made projections of the future course of the epidemic more difficult.

The sensitivity of the surveillance case definition for capturing information on [fatal] HIV-associated disease has increased with each revision and is estimated to be more than 90 percent, [but still reflects variations in diagnostic practices.] In some instances, severe, life-threatening conditions in HIV-infected individuals, such as bacterial and unspecified pneumonias, may still not meet the case definition, or a person with an AIDS-indicator disease may not have been tested for HIV.[7] For example, one hospital in New York City reported that if an HIV test result had been available for all suspect AIDS cases, the number of AIDS cases reported

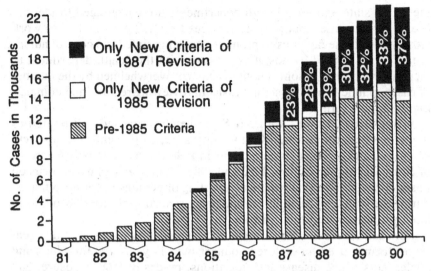

FIGURE 8-1.   AIDS cases in the United States by half-year of diagnosis (adjusted for reporting delay) and category of case definition, July 1981 to December 1990.

from that hospital might have increased 40 percent during 1988.[8] This finding led to a change in procedures at that hospital that increased the availability of HIV testing.

The CDC is considering a further expansion of the AIDS surveillance case definition, which would include HIV-infected persons with a CD4+ lymphocyte count less than 200/μl. CD4+ lymphocytes are the primary target of HIV and decline progressively throughout the course of HIV infection. Their level is used as a marker of clinical status and prognosis and as a guide to the administration of antiretroviral and prophylactic therapies. This expansion would include many persons earlier in the course of HIV infection compared with the 1987 reporting criteria, many with illnesses not encompassed by the 1987 reporting criteria, and those at highest risk for progression to severe morbidity.

Data Collection

All fifty states, the District of Columbia, Puerto Rico, the Virgin Islands, Guam, and the Pacific Trust territories require reporting of AIDS cases to state or local health departments. The CDC has developed guidelines to assist health departments in stimulating AIDS case reporting and has encouraged them to take an active rather than a passive approach to AIDS surveillance.[9] Through surveillance-cooperative agreements supported by the CDC, state and local health departments are encouraged to identify health care facilities that provide services to AIDS patients and to work closely with these facilities to promote reporting. Infection control nurses are often designated by hospitals to work with the health department to facilitate reporting; in some facilities that are overwhelmed by the number of cases, public health personnel assist in reviewing records and completing the report forms.

Increasingly, persons with AIDS are being diagnosed and treated as outpatients. In the Seattle–King County area, 25 percent of cases were diagnosed and reported as outpatients in 1988 compared to only 6 percent of cases diagnosed between 1982 and 1985.[10] Thus, an exclusive focus on hospital-based reporting will miss reporting of persons never hospitalized during the course of their illness and delay reporting of those hospitalized later in the course of their disease.

For each case identified, a standard case report form is used. A different report form is used for children younger than 13 years and for adults and adolescents, since disease manifestations, modes of HIV exposure, and laboratory diagnoses in children vary from those in adults and adolescents. In addition, because perinatal (mother-to-infant) transmission of HIV is the predominant mode of exposure among children with AIDS, the pediatric form collects information on the risk of the mother. Cases are reported by name to the state health department and by an alpha-numeric code called "Soundex" to the CDC; Soundex codes assist in protecting confidentiality since a Soundex code cannot be converted back to a patient's name. Soundex codes and dates of birth are used to identify duplicate reports submitted by states. Most states submit their data monthly to the CDC via a computer diskette.

Analysis of Data

AIDS surveillance data are routinely tabulated by date of report. Because the median time from HIV infection to development of AIDS is approximately 10 years, trends in AIDS cases may be monitored using broad time periods. For example, the surveillance report that is issued monthly provides data comparing the most recent 12-month period to the previous 12-month period.

Analyses by date of diagnosis give a more accurate description of trends, being less dependent on reporting fluctuations; however, delays in reporting have a substantial impact on the number of cases diagnosed and reported in recent time periods. Ten to twenty percent of cases may be reported more than 1 year after diagnosis. In addition, delays vary by geographic region, exposure category, and age. Reporting delays can be estimated and data adjusted accordingly to estimate the number of cases that are likely to be diagnosed during a given period of time.[11, 12]

Projections of the course of the HIV epidemic are critical for developing public health policies for planning future prevention efforts and to anticipate health care needs. Almost all mathematical models that project the future course of the epidemic have relied on AIDS surveillance data, and such data will, for the immediate future, continue to be critical for predicting the future course of the epidemic. Currently, one of the most widely used methods for short-term projections ("back-calculation") uses AIDS incidence data together with information on the distribution of the incubation period. These data are used to reconstruct the number of persons who must have been previously infected to account for the previously observed AIDS cases and to estimate the future number of cases. These methods must be refined, particularly as effective therapy becomes available that may alter the incubation period.

Dissemination of Data

Data are disseminated widely by the CDC. Monthly surveillance reports are issued that provide tabulations of data for states and major metropolitan areas, with breakdowns by age, sex, race, and exposure categories. Data are also provided monthly to a national telecommunication network used by the Public Health Foundation and to the public via a recorded message on a toll-free telephone line. Data that cannot be used to identify individuals are also released at least twice a year via a public use data tape, diskettes, and a detailed set of microfiche tables, which include summary data on individual states and major metropolitan areas.[13]

State and local health departments also provide data to their reporting sources, including physicians and infection control practitioners, through published monthly or quarterly reports. Some health departments provide confidential data specific to an individual health care provider (e.g., a report for a hospital contrasting its reported cases with county or statewide data). AIDS data are also used for presentations to policymakers, clinicians, the news media, and the general public.

Evaluation

Most evaluations of AIDS surveillance have focused on completeness and timeliness of reporting.[14, 15] As part of the cooperative agreements between the CDC and the local and state health departments, AIDS data must be evaluated for completeness and timeliness. At a minimum, most areas use death certificate reviews as an evaluation tool; areas that find many cases initially through death certificate review are advised that surveillance activities may need to be strengthened.

Review of hospital discharge data has also been useful. A study in South Carolina conducted for 1986 and early 1987 established that about 40 percent of persons hospitalized with disease meeting the AIDS case definition had not been reported to the health department.[16] Following the study, regular contacts between the hospitals and the health department were initiated and a subsequent study documented an improvement in completeness of reporting, with 93 percent of hospitalized AIDS patients reported. Oregon, which initially had a similar level of underreporting before 1987, estimated 95 percent completeness of reporting after surveillance activities were strengthened.[17] As of May 1988 all states and U.S. territories were funded to improve their surveillance activities for AIDS.[18] Overall, completeness of reporting of diagnosed AIDS cases is estimated to be 80 to 90 percent nationwide.[19]

Delays in reporting are quite variable and depend on the strength of the surveillance system and the public health ties with the clinical community. About half of all cases in 1989 were reported within 3 months of diagnosis, with about 15 percent reported more than 1 year after diagnosis. Delays are particularly long for pediatric cases and for transfusion-associated cases. Although delays can occur at any point in the process, it is the time between diagnosis and report to the state or local health department that is most lengthy. The time between report to the local or state health department to the CDC has generally been less than 1 month, as has the time from receipt of data to analysis and dissemination.

USE OF EXISTING DATA SYSTEMS

In addition to AIDS case surveillance, other data are needed to determine the impact of HIV disease. For example, vital statistics data have been used to demonstrate that HIV/AIDS has become a leading cause of death in the United States in young adult men and women.[20, 21]

Other data have also been useful in establishing the spectrum of disease manifestations associated with HIV infection. For example, analysis of vital statistics has demonstrated that an increase in deaths from pneumonia, blood disorders, and other causes has been associated with the increase in AIDS.[20] An evaluation of hospital records of a sample of intravenous drug users who died in New York City between 1981 and 1986 established that many of these deaths may be attributable to HIV infection but did not meet the AIDS surveillance case definition.[7] Hospital discharge data can also be used to determine the burden of HIV disease on health care services; Medicaid records, health maintenance organization records, insurance records, and registries for drugs can all be used to provide a more complete picture of health care service utilization for HIV.[22]

SEROPREVALENCE SURVEYS

Two types of surveys are used to monitor levels and trends of HIV infection in the United States: blinded and nonblinded.[23] In blinded surveys, blood specimens that are usually collected for other purposes are tested for HIV only after personal identifiers are removed. Such surveys were initiated to decrease self-selection bias. A blinded survey of sexually transmitted disease patients in Albuquerque, New Mexico, found the rate of HIV infection among the 82 percent of patients who agreed to participate in nonblinded testing to be five times less than the rate among the 18 percent who were tested only in a blinded fashion.[24] Eliminating personally identifying information avoids the need for informed consent and minimizes participation bias. In nonblinded serosurveys, persons who have consented to HIV testing are interviewed extensively regarding HIV risk. This type of survey evaluates the patterns of HIV transmission, while the blinded surveys quantify the prevalence of infection.

To facilitate rapid and consistent implementation of surveys across the United States, the CDC established cooperative agreements in 44 major metropolitan areas in 1987 to 1989 to conduct blinded surveys in various clinical settings, including sexually transmitted disease clinics, drug treatment centers, women's health clinics, tuberculosis clinics, and sentinel hospitals, and in childbearing women.[25] Nonblinded surveys complement blinded surveys by providing more extensive information on specific risk behaviors in settings with appreciable levels of infection, especially sexually transmitted disease clinics and drug treatment centers. Serologic testing of patients with tuberculosis is also increasing since tuberculosis may present clinically as an opportunistic disease in persons with HIV infection.

In addition to surveys targeted at clinical settings, studies are underway of data from several large segments of the population with routine HIV testing, including blood donors, military applicants, active-duty military personnel, and Job Corps entrants. Risk information is systematically collected on HIV-positive donors, a population that excludes self-reported homosexual and bisexual men, IV drug users, and persons with hemophilia. Prevalence is documented in first-time donors, and prevalence and incidence of new infection are observed in repeat donors. Civilian applicants for military service have been screened serologically since October 1985 and active-duty military have been screened periodically since 1986, directly indicating the annual incidence of HIV infection in this population.[26] Information on Job Corps entrants (disadvantaged youths 16 to 21 years old) has been important in assessing trends in HIV infection in young persons, particularly those from inner-city minority groups.

Blinded testing of blood specimens of newborn infants has been implemented in most surveys by using filter-paper blood specimens that had been obtained by heel-stick puncture for routine, metabolic screening[27, 28]; positive tests reflect the presence of maternal antibody, but not necessarily infection of the newborn (only about one-third of infants testing positive at birth actually acquire infection from their infected mother). This survey approach provides information on the prevalence of infection among women delivering live-born infants and also provides the basis for estimating the number of infants infected through perinatal transmission annually.

The geographic differences in prevalence of HIV infection make seroprevalence surveys particularly useful in areas with a substantial number of persons at high risk (e.g., intravenous drug users) but a low prevalence of HIV infection. An increase in prevalence over time can serve as an early warning that the transmission of HIV is increasing in particular populations, and this information can be disseminated immediately to target prevention activities.

In order to get a direct estimate of the number of HIV infections in the country, a survey was designed by the CDC based on a probability sample of households throughout the country. The study design called for 50,000 respondents between 18 and 54 years of age. The pilot phase was completed, with field studies in Pittsburgh and Dallas. In this phase, the feasibility of such a survey was evaluated, with attempts made to measure the impact of people at risk selectively declining participation. After careful review of the findings of the pilot phase, a decision was made not to conduct the full national survey.

HIV REPORTING

Since the development of diagnostic tests for HIV infection, health agencies have struggled with the issue of whether persons with HIV infection should be reported to health departments. Many are concerned that HIV reporting by name may deter individuals from being tested (i.e., individuals may fear that HIV test results may be disclosed and discrimination may occur). Others, noting that the risk of breaking confidentiality is remote, have cited multiple benefits of HIV reporting.

HIV-reporting data have been used to alert public health professionals to geographic areas in which HIV transmission has not been detected through AIDS surveillance.[30] In addition, these data provide a minimum estimate of the number of persons known to be infected with HIV. Since all infected persons require some level of health care, this information may be useful for planning current and future health care services. Because HIV-infection reports depend upon testing practices rather than on persons seeking medical care for an illness, trends in these reports must be interpreted more cautiously than AIDS surveillance data; trends in HIV infection reporting may reflect trends in testing patterns rather than in HIV incidence. Thus, to monitor the HIV epidemic, data from HIV infection reporting can complement but cannot be substituted for AIDS surveillance and HIV serosurveys.

The potential benefits of HIV-infection reporting may be most fully realized in providing a framework for implementing and evaluating prevention and early intervention activities. South Carolina has used HIV-infection reports as a framework for their partner notification activities, which provide direct counseling and health education to infected and exposed individuals.[31] They have demonstrated the ability of partner notification to identify persons who previously did not know they were infected, and they have documented changes in behavior following counseling. More recently, following the release of recommendations in 1989 to treat many asymptomatic HIV-infected individuals with antiretroviral therapy, some states have considered use of HIV reporting by name to assure that patients have access to appropriate medical follow-up. For example, HIV-infection reporting has been used by some states to link individuals to early intervention services, such as testing of immune function.

Since 1985, when testing for HIV-infection status first became feasible, an increasing number of states have required HIV-infection reporting, but the requirements for reporting have varied considerably among states.[32] Some states do not require reporting by name. Other states require reporting by name but support anonymous testing and counseling sites, and therefore have incomplete reporting of persons who have tested positive for HIV. Most states that adopted a reporting-by-name requirement in the 1980s are those in which the incidence of AIDS has been relatively low. Because the HIV-reporting systems among the states have been developed independently, the information they collect also varies. The CDC has been working with those states adopting HIV-infection reporting to develop a uniform system of reporting to allow comparison of data from one area to another.

SUMMARY

Over the first decade of the AIDS epidemic, the concept of HIV and AIDS surveillance has broadened considerably. Tracking the morbidity and mortality related to HIV, following the characteristics of those affected, determining the prevalence and incidence of HIV infection, targeting and evaluating prevention activities, and projecting the future course of the epidemic have been the objectives of HIV/AIDS surveillance. No one system has been able to meet all of these objectives. Data from AIDS surveillance, the "family" of serosurveys, and other data systems such as those involving vital statistics and hospital discharge data comprise an information system stronger than any one of its component parts.

Notes

1. Jaffe, H. W., K. Choi, P. A. Thomas et al. 1983. National case-control study of Kaposi's sarcoma and *Pneumocystis carinii* pneumonia in homosexual men: epidemiologic results. *Ann Intern Med* 99:293.
2. Centers for Disease Control. 1990. Estimates of HIV prevalence and projected AIDS cases: summary of a workshop. *MMWR* 39:110–119.
3. Selik, R. M., H. W. Haverkos, and J. W. Curran. 1984. Acquired immune deficiency syndrome (AIDS) trends in the United States, 1978–1982. *Am J Med* 76:493–500.
4. Centers for Disease Control. 1985. Revision of the case definition of acquired immunodeficiency syndrome for national reporting: United States. *MMWR* 34:373–375.
5. Centers for Disease Control. 1987. Revision of the CDC surveillance case definition for acquired immunodeficiency syndrome. *MMWR* 36(1S):1S–15S.
6. Selik, R. M., J. W. Buehler, J. M. Karon, M. E. Chamberland, and R. L. Berkelman. 1990. Impact of the 1987 revision of the case definition of acquired immune deficiency syndrome in the United States. *J AIDS* 3:73–82.
7. Stoneburner, R. L., D. C. Des Jarlais, D. Benezra et al. 1988. A larger spectrum of severe HIV-1-related disease in intravenous drug users in New York City. *Science* 242:916–918.
8. Masterson, A., A. Oppermann, and S. Landesman. 1989. Marked underreporting of CDC-defined AIDS due to poor utilization of the HIV antibody test. Abstract in: *Abstracts of the V International Conference on AIDS,* 55. Montreal, Quebec: International Development Research Centre, Health and Welfare Canada, World Health Organization.
9. Centers for Disease Control. 1989. *Acquired Immunodeficiency Syndrome (AIDS) Surveillance Guidelines.* Atlanta, Ga.: CDC.
10. Hopkins, S., W. Lafferty, J. Honey, and M. Hurlich. 1989. Trends in the outpatient diagnosis of AIDS: implications for epidemiologic analysis and surveillance. Abstracts in: *Abstracts of the V International Conference on AIDS,* 111. Montreal, Quebec: International Development Research Centre, Health and Welfare Canada, World Health Organization.
11. Karon, J. M., O. J. Devine, and W. M. Morgan. 1989. Predicting AIDS incidence by extrapolating from recent trends. In: *Mathematical and Statistical Approaches to AIDS Epidemiology: Lecture Notes in Biomathematics,* vol. 83, Castillo-Chavex, C., ed. Berlin: Springer-Verlag, 58–88.
12. Centers for Disease Control. 1990. Update: acquired immunodeficiency syndrome: United States, 1989. *MMWR* 39:81–86.

13. Centers for Disease Control. 1989. *Acquired Immunodeficiency Syndrome (AIDS) Public Information Data Set.* Atlanta, Ga.: CDC.
14. Hardy, A. M., E. T. Starcher, W. M. Morgan et al. 1987. Review of death certificates to assess completeness of AIDS case reporting. *Public Health Rep* 102:386–391.
15. Chamberland, M. E., J. R. Allen, J. M. Monroe et al. 1985. Acquired immunodeficiency syndrome in New York City: evaluation of an active surveillance system. *JAMA* 254:383–387.
16. Conway, G. A., B. Colley-Niemeyer, C. Pursley et al. 1989. Underreporting of AIDS cases in South Carolina, 1986 and 1987. *JAMA* 262:2859–2863.
17. Modesitt, S., S. Hulman, and D. Fleming. 1990. Evaluation of active versus passive AIDS surveillance in Oregon. *Am J Public Health* 80:463–464.
18. Buehler, J. W., R. L. Berkelman, and J. W. Curran. 1989. Reporting of AIDS: tracking HIV morbidity and mortality. *JAMA* 262:2896–2897.
19. Buehler, J. W., R. L. Berkelman, and J. K. Stehr-Green. In press. The completeness of AIDS surveillance. *J AIDS.*
20. Buehler, J. W., O. Devine, R. L. Berkelman, and F. Chevarley. 1990. Impact of HIV epidemic on mortality trends in men 25–44 years of age: United States. *Am J Public Health* 80:1080–1085.
21. Chu, S., J. W. Buehler, R. Berkelman. 1990. Impact of the human immunodeficiency virus epidemic on mortality in women of reproductive age: United States. *JAMA* 264:225–229.
22. Lafferty, W. E., S. G. Hopkins, J. Honey et al. 1988. Hospital charges for people with AIDS in Washington State: utilization of a statewide hospital discharge data base. *Am J Public Health* 78:949–952.
23. Dondero, Jr., T. J., M. Pappaioanou, and J. W. Curran. 1988. Monitoring the levels and trends of HIV infection: the Public Health Service's HIV surveillance program. *Public Health Rep* 103:213–220.
24. Hull, H. F., C. J. Bettinger, M. M. Gallaher et al. 1988. Comparison of HIV antibody prevalence in patients consenting to and declining HIV antibody testing in an STD clinic. *JAMA* 260:935–938.
25. Pappaioanou, M., Dondero, T. J. Jr., L. R. Peterson et al. 1990. The family of HIV seroprevalence surveys: objectives, methods, and uses of sentinel surveillance for HIV in the United States. *Public Health Rep* 105:113–119.
26. McNeil, J. G., J. F. Brundage, Z. F. Wann, D. S. Burke, R. N. Miller, and the Walter-Reed Retrovirus Research Group. 1989. Direct measurement of human immunodeficiency virus seroconversion in a serially tested population of young adults in the United States Army, October 1985 to October 1987. *NEJM* 320:1581–1585.
27. Pappaioanou, M., J. R. George, W. H. Hannon et al. 1990. HIV seroprevalence surveys of childbearing women: objectives, methods, and uses of the data. *Public Health Rep* 105:147–152.
28. Hoff, R., V. P. Beradi, B. J. Weiblem et al. 1988. Seroprevalence of human immunodeficiency virus among childbearing women: estimation by testing samples of blood from newborns. *NEJM* 318:525–530.

29. Novick, L. F., D. Berns, R. Stricof et al. 1989. HIV seroprevalence in newborns in New York State. *JAMA* 261:1745–1750.
30. Hoffman, R. E., S. E. Valway, F. C. Wolf et al. 1989. Comparison of AIDS and HIV antibody surveillance data in Colorado. *J AIDS* 2:194–200.
31. Wykoff, R. F., C. W. Heath, S. L. Hollis et al. Contact tracing to identify human immunodeficiency virus infection in a rural community. *JAMA* 259:3563–3566.
32. Centers for Disease Control. 1990. Surveillance for HIV infection: United States. *MMWR* 39:853, 859–861.

9

The Surveillance of Nosocomial Infections

Robert P. Gaynes

Since the beginning of organized infection control programs, surveillance has been advocated as essential for recognizing nosocomial infection problems and for developing effective prevention measures.[1, 2] Its efficacy in helping to reduce nosocomial infections has been reported by several investigators[3-7] and supported by organizations that set standards of care within hospitals, such as the American Hospital Association, the Joint Commission on Accreditation of Healthcare Organizations (JCAHO), and the Health Care Financing Administration.[8-10]

Surveillance of nosocomial infections differs little from surveillance in other settings, with perhaps two exceptions. First, epidemiologists in the hospital setting are often called upon to act when surveillance determines an increase of a very small number of cases, such as two or three wound infections in a month caused by the same bacterium. Second, and perhaps more important, surveillance of nosocomial infections differs from surveillance in the community because so much information is routinely documented in a hospital, such as the times of procedures and the persons who were involved. This allows retrospective epidemiologic studies to be performed with a degree of accuracy that is not possible in most other settings.

CONTEMPORARY INFLUENCES

Several factors have influenced the current practices of surveillance of nosocomial infections. Perhaps the three most important have been the JCAHO recommendations, the Study on Efficacy of Nosocomial Infection Control (SENIC), and the introduction of Diagnostic-Related Groups

121

(DRGs). The JCAHO established infection surveillance as a function of the medical staff in 1964.[11] Although the recommendations changed over the years, the JCAHO provided the structure and force for the surveillance of nosocomial infections in U.S. hospitals. The scientific basis for surveillance of nosocomial infections was provided by the SENIC study, published in 1985.[3] This study found that the hospitals with strong surveillance components in their infection control programs were more effective in reducing nosocomial infections at virtually all of its sites than those with programs that did not devote efforts to surveillance. Finally, additional motivation for surveillance of nosocomial infections has come from the introduction of DRGs into U.S. hospitals for reimbursement of care. The DRGs allow for a single payment to a hospital for a discharge diagnosis; for example, inguinal hernia repair. If a nosocomial infection occurs, the hospital loses money either because no further money was allowed or the additional money for the complication (the infection) was insufficient to cover the hospital's cost for care. Thus, with the introduction of DRGs, the hospital administration had a monetary impetus to establish an effective infection control program. Surveillance became one of its essential components.[12]

METHODS OF SURVEILLANCE OF NOSOCOMIAL INFECTIONS

A method for conducting surveillance was generally not available until 1969, when the Centers for Disease Control (CDC) reported its first surveillance study of nosocomial infections.[13] This and subsequent studies have outlined the four major sites of nosocomial infection (and their approximate percentages): urinary tract infections (40 percent), surgical wound infections (18 percent), nosocomial pneumonia (17 percent), and primary bloodstream infections (7 percent). Other infections make up 18 percent of nosocomial infections. However, major variations in these percentages occur depending upon the type of hospital, patient-related factors, methodologic problems related to the identification of nosocomial infections, and data collection techniques. The latter can affect the reliability of the data and make comparisons among the hospitals difficult. They include a wide variation among observers in determining infections, the lack of bacteriologic documentation of infections, and a lack of adherence to surveillance protocol. While these problems have not been completely solved, progress has been made in infection control and surveillance; standard definitions for nosocomial infections are available and widely used, hospitals are required to have a trained individual to perform surveillance, and the use of bacteriologic tests by physicians to diagnose nosocomial infections has increased substantially.[14-16]

TABLE 9-1   Methods of Surveillance of Nosocomial Infections

1. Hospitalwide Surveillance
2. Targeted Surveillance
    a. Unit-directed surveillance (e.g., intensive care unit)
    b. Site-directed surveillance (e.g., bloodstream infections)
    c. Rotating surveillance

The precise method for surveillance of nosocomial infections remains controversial. No one method is appropriate for all hospitals, and must vary depending upon the characteristics of the hospital, the type of patients in the hospital, the resources available for surveillance, and the types of nosocomial infections occurring in the hospital.

The initial approach to surveillance of nosocomial infections involves the events and the cohort of patients to be monitored. The CDC definitions for nosocomial infections are now widely used, although some modifications may be needed in individual hospitals.[15] The choice of the cohort of patients to monitor is basically a choice between hospitalwide surveillance or targeted surveillance (Table 9-1) While many hospitals continue to perform hospitalwide surveillance, most recognize its limited usefulness for assessing the quality of patient care.[17] Whether the overall hospital infection rate is useful has been the subject of controversy.[18, 19] Because an overall rate does not account for the contribution of risk factors to infections, it is too insensitive to be useful for assessing the quality of patient care or the effectiveness of intervention measures. Therefore, many practitioners choose targeted surveillance for their approach.

Once these decisions have been made, the issue of case finding appears. There is great debate over the most sensitive, specific, and efficient method of finding cases of nosocomial infection, and the methods used vary widely.[20] However, whatever the initial "red flagging" method used (e.g., review of microbiology cultures, temperature charts of patients, etc.), a thorough review of the patient's medical record is essential to achieving adequate sensitivity and specificity in determining nearly all nosocomial infections.

Once the data on nosocomial infections have been collected, the acquisition of denominator data is necessary. The need to calculate rates is a hallmark of any surveillance program, but in this instance, the choice of denominators is critical for producing rates for inter- or intrahospital comparison.[21] The use of the number of patient days is generally preferable to the number of patients (admissions or discharges) for the denominator if overall infection rates are calculated, since the former at least partially controls for the average length of hospital stay, which is a confounding variable for most nosocomial infections. However, rates that use these numbers in the denominator fail to control for variations in exposure to medical devices, which are major risk factors for most nosocomial infections.[22] Recording and analyzing data on patients with nosocomial infections generally requires a computer unless the size of the hospital is very small; that is, less than 100 beds.

THE NATIONAL NOSOCOMIAL INFECTIONS SURVEILLANCE SYSTEM

With the controversy surrounding the best method for surveillance, some guidance has been provided by the CDC's National Nosocomial Infections Surveillance (NNIS) system. The trends in the approach to surveillance of nosocomial infection are reflected in the history of the NNIS system. NNIS began in 1970 when selected U.S. hospitals routinely reported their nosocomial infection surveillance data for aggregation into a national database. It is currently the only source of national data on the epidemiology of nosocomial infections in the United States. Before 1986, all surveillance performed in the NNIS system was hospitalwide. However, as targeted surveillance became more popular, NNIS personnel developed additional surveillance components to serve as more efficient methods of surveillance.

Description of NNIS Methodology

Hospitals participating in the NNIS system provide general medical–surgical inpatient services to adults or children requiring acute care. The identities of the 119 hospitals currently participating in NNIS are confidential.[22]

All NNIS data are collected using four standardized protocols, called surveillance components; hospitalwide (the only component available until October 1986), adult and pediatric intensive care unit (ICU), high-risk nursery (HRN), and surgical patient. All infections are categorized into major and specific infection sites using standard CDC definitions that include laboratory and clinical criteria.[14]

1. *Hospitalwide surveillance component.* Infection control practitioners (ICP) using this component collect nosocomial infection data on all patients at all sites of infection. Infection rates may be calculated by service using hospital discharges or patient days.

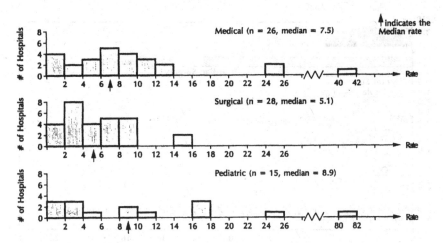

FIGURE 9-1.   Central intravenous catheter–associated bloodstream infection rates per 1,000 central intravenous catheter days, by type of intensive care unit, NNIS, 1987–1989.

2. *Adult and pediatric intensive care unit surveillance component.* ICP collect data on nosocomial infections in patients located in ICU(s) and ICU-specific denominator data. Site-specific infection rates can be calculated based on the appropriate denominator—for instance, the number of patients at risk—using such factors as total patient days, days of indwelling urinary catheterization, central vascular cannulation, or ventilator assistance.

3. *High-risk nursery surveillance component.* ICP collect data on nosocomial infections in patients located in HRN(s) and HRN-specific denominator data. Site-specific infection rates can be calculated using the number of patients at risk, total patient days, days of umbilical catheter/ central line use, and days of ventilator assistance for each birthweight category.

4. *Surgical patient surveillance component.*

   a. Detailed Option. In the detailed option, the hospital personnel select from the NNIS operative procedure list the procedures they wish to follow. ICP collect data on nosocomial infections in surgical patients for the selected operations.

   b. Limited Option. Using this option, all patients undergoing all NNIS operative procedures are monitored for infections. The denominator data are the number of times each NNIS operative procedure was performed and the total number of NNIS operative procedures in each traditional wound class.

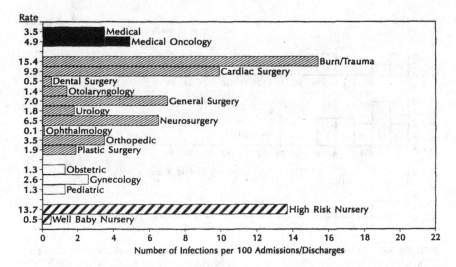

FIGURE 9-2.   Overall nosocomial infection rates, by service and subspecialty, NNIS Hospitals, 1987–1989.

The rationale for the development of the components for targeted surveillance was primarily efficiency. For example, previous studies in intensive care units found that ICU patients had disproportionately more nosocomial infections at all sites. In one hospital, the infection rate in the ICU was three times higher (18 percent) than in general medical–surgical patients.[23] This hospital found that 33 to 45 percent of the bloodstream infections occurred in patients in the intensive care unit, although these patients occupied only 8 percent of the beds.[24] By using the ICU component, hospitals are able to monitor patients who have devices that are associated with high infection risks (see Fig. 9-1) These device-specific rates appear to lend themselves to interhospital comparison more than an overall infection rate. One hospital participating in the NNIS system used the ICU component to identify high infection rates associated with the use of certain devices, and was able to measure a reduction in device-specific infection rates in the ICU after the institution of changes in patient care practices.[25]

The HRN surveillance component was developed because studies have shown that neonates in the HRN are among the most susceptible to nosocomial infections[26, 27] (see Fig. 9-2). Bloodstream infections occur frequently; the sepsis rate in one HRN was 4 percent, and in another, 13 percent.[28, 29] In ways similar to the ICU component, the device-specific infection rates appear to be the most useful for interhospital comparison.[30]

The surgical patient component is based on the findings of the SENIC project that patients who undergo surgical operations are three times more likely to develop a nosocomial infection than nonsurgical patients,[31] and that surveillance is effective in reducing the surgical wound infection rate, particularly when surgeon-specific infection rates are fed back to surgeons.[32, 33] A risk index that was a better predictor of surgical wound infection (SWI) risk than wound class alone was demonstrated in the SENIC project.[34] An NNIS infection risk index has confirmed the findings of the SENIC project and extended them to an analysis of wound infection risk by procedure.[35]

The NNIS system has certain limitations. The intensity of the surveillance efforts varies in that there are different sources used for case finding, different amounts of infection control resources, including staffing, and a variable frequency of culturing and other diagnostic tests, including the availability of tests such as viral cultures. Finally, no consistent method for post-discharge surveillance exists in NNIS hospitals, although approximately one-third have some method of post-discharge surveillance.

The lessons learned from 20 years of surveillance from the NNIS system have proved useful for advising hospitals on effective methods for conducting surveillance of nosocomial infections. These methods are also potentially useful for assessing other noninfectious outcomes of hospital care.

If comparative surveillance data are to be at least useful for assessing the quality of care in U.S. hospitals, the same surveillance methods must be used and the intrinsic susceptibility of patients must be controlled.[36] The NNIS components were in part developed to address these issues. However, the infection control community must meet the challenge to determine how surveillance data can be used to evaluate and influence hospital practices and to develop more effective strategies to prevent nosocomial infections.

Notes

1. Brachman, P. S. 1963. Surveillance of institutionally acquired infections. *Proceedings of the National Conference on Institutionally Acquired Infections*, September 4–16, 138–147. Department of Health, Education, and Welfare, United States Public Health Service.
2. Eickhoff, T. C. 1967. Hospital infection control begins with good surveillance. *JAHA* 41:118–120.
3. Haley, R. W., D. H. Culver, J. W. White et al. 1985. The efficacy of infection surveillance and control programs in preventing nosocomial infections in U.S. hospitals. *Am J Epidemiol* 121:182–205.
4. Shoji, K. T., K. Axnick, and M. W. Rytel. 1974. Infections and antibiotic use in a large municipal hospital 1970–1972: a prospective analysis of the effectiveness of a continuous surveillance program. *Health Lab Sciences* 11:283–292.

5. Brewer, G. E. 1915. Studies in aseptic technique, with a report of some recent observations at the Roosevelt Hospital. *JAMA* 64:1369–1372.
6. Olson, M., M. O'Connor, and M. L. Schwartz. 1984. Surgical wound infections: A five-year prospective study of 20,193 wounds at the Minneapolis VA Medical Center. *Ann Surg* 199:253–259.
7. Cruse, P. J. E., and R. Foord. 1973. A five-year prospective study of 23,649 surgical wounds. *Arch Surg* 107:206–210.
8. American Hospital Association. 1958. Prevention and control of *Staphylococcus* infections in hospitals. In: U.S. Public Health Service—Communicable Disease Center and National Academy of Sciences— National Research Council. *Proceedings of the National Conference on Hospital-Acquired Staphylococcal Disease*, XII–XXVI. Atlanta, Ga: Communicable Disease Center.
9. Joint Commission on Accreditation of Healthcare Organizations. 1976. *Accreditation Manual for Hospitals, 1976*. Chicago: JCAHO.
10. Health Care Financing Administration. 1986. Condition of participation: infection control. 42CFR 482.42. *Federal Register* June 17, 51:22010:485–553.
11. Joint Commission on Accreditation of Healthcare Organizations. 1964. *Standards for Hospital Accreditation*. Chicago: JCAHO.
12. Haley, R. W., J. W. White, D. H. Culver, and J. M. Hughes. 1987. The financial incentive for hospitals to prevent nosocomial infections under the prospective payment system. *JAMA* 257:1611–1614.
13. Eickhoff, T. C., P. S. Brachman, J. V. Bennett, and J. Brown. 1969. Surveillance of nosocomial infections in community hospitals. I. Surveillance methods, effectiveness and initial results. *J Infect Dis* 120:305–317.
14. Garner, J. S., W. R. Jarvis, T. C. Horan et al. 1988. CDC definitions of nosocomial infections: 1988. *Am J Med* 16:128–140.
15. Joint Commission on Accreditation of Healthcare Organizations. 1989. *Accreditation Manual for Hospitals, 1990*. Chicago: JCAHO.
16. Haley, R. W., D. H. Culver, W. M. Morgan et al. 1985. Increased recognition of infectious diseases in U.S. hospitals through increased use of diagnostic tests, 1970–1976. *Am J Epidemiol* 121:168–180.
17. Haley, R. W. 1985. Surveillance by objective: a new priority-directed approach to the control of nosocomial infections. *Am J Infect Control* 13:78–89.
18. Larson, E. 1980. A comparison of methods for surveillance of nosocomial infections. *Infect Control* 1:377–380.
19. Fuchs, P. C. 1987. Will the real infection rate please stand? *Infect Control* 8:235–236.
20. Freeman, J., and J. E. McGowan, Jr. 1981. Methodologic issues in hospital epidemiology: rates, case-finding, and interpretation. *Rev Infect Dis* 3:658–667.
21. Edwards, J. E., W. R. Jarvis, D. H. Culver et al. 1991. Nosocomial infection rates in adult and pediatric intensive care units in the United States. *Am J Med* 91(3B):185s–191s.
22. Emori, T. G., D. H. Culver, T. C. Horan et al. 1991. The National Nosocomial

Infections Surveillance system: description of methodology. *Am J Infect Control* 19:19–35.

23. Donowitz, L. G., R. P. Wenzel, and J. W. Hoyt. 1982. High risk of hospital-acquired infection in the ICU patient. *Crit Care Med* 10:355–357.
24. Wenzel, R., C. A. Osterman, and L. Donowitz. 1981. Identification of procedure-related nosocomial infections in high-risk patients. *Rev Infect Dis* 3:701–707.
25. Selva, J., C. Toledo, A. Maroney, and S. Forlenza. 1989. The value of participation in the CDC's National Nosocomial Infections Surveillance (NNIS) system in a large teaching hospital. Paper presented at the APIC Sixteenth Annual Educational Conference.
26. Hemming, V. G., J. C. Overall, Jr., and M. R. Britt. 1976. Nosocomial infections in a newborn intensive-care unit. *NEJM* 294:1310–1316.
27. Goldmann, D. A., W. A. Durbin, and J. Freeman. 1981. Nosocomial infections in a neonatal intensive care unit. *J Infect Dis* 144:449–459.
28. Townsend, T. R., and R. P. Wenzel. 1981. Nosocomial bloodstream infections in a newborn intensive care unit. *Am J Epidemiol* 114:73–80.
29. Kotloff, K. L., L. R. Blackmon, and J. H. Tenney. 1989. Nosocomial sepsis in the neonatal intensive care unit. *Southern Med J* 82:699–704.
30. Gaynes, R. P., D. H. Culver, W. J. Martone et al. 1991. Comparison of nosocomial infection rates in neonatal intensive care units in the United States. *Am J Med* 91(3B):193s–196s.
31. Haley, R. W., T. M. Hooton, and D. H. Culver. 1981. Nosocomial infections in U.S. hospitals, 1975–1976. *Am J Med* 70:947–959.
32. Cruse, P. J. E. 1981. Wound infection surveillance. *Rev Infect Dis* 3:734–737.
33. Haley, R. W., D. H. Culver, J. W. White et al. 1985. The efficacy of infection surveillance and control programs in preventing nosocomial infections in U.S. hospitals. *Am J Epidemiol* 121:182–205.
34. Haley, R. W., D. H. Culver, W. M. Morgan et al. 1985. Identifying patients at high risk of surgical wound infection. *Am J Epidemiol* 121:206–215.
35. Culver, D. H., T. C. Horan, R. P. Gaynes et al. 1991. Surgical wound infection rates by wound class, operative procedure, and patient risk index. *Am J Med* 91(3B):152s–157s.
36. Larson, E., L. F. Oram, and E. Hedrick. 1988. Nosocomial infection rates as an indicator of quality. *Med. Care* 26:676–684.

10

Chronic Disease Surveillance

Paul L. Garbe and Stephen B. Blount

Increasingly, the principles of disease surveillance have been applied to a variety of chronic conditions, thus extending beyond their original purpose of guiding local, state, and national infectious disease programs.[1] Excluding conditions related to infancy, six categories of chronic disease are among the ten leading causes of death and years of potential life lost before age 65: heart diseases, malignant neoplasms, cerebrovascular diseases, chronic liver diseases and cirrhosis, chronic obstructive pulmonary diseases, and diabetes mellitus.[2, 3] Although chronic disease surveillance efforts are relatively new at the local and state levels, they will become even more important as the number of older Americans—with their increased need for chronic disease care—escalates dramatically over the coming decades.

CHARACTERISTICS OF CHRONIC DISEASE SURVEILLANCE SYSTEMS

Chronic disease surveillance systems historically have focused on population-based summaries of disease patterns rather than the case- or event-based reporting systems used in notifiable disease surveillance systems. Important early activities for chronic disease surveillance are to establish baseline information and to follow up with ongoing examination and summarization of temporal trends and geographic patterns in chronic disease occurrence. Systematic chronic disease surveillance allows us to identify changing risk groups and to examine disparities in disease burden and access to medical care. It also enables us to detect geographic patterns of disease so that we can better target intervention and control programs.

130

For instance, a state health department, faced with scarce resources, may use a surveillance system to identify communities with the highest cancer incidence or mortality rates, and then establish cancer control programs only in those communities. Finally, surveillance helps us to assess and monitor comorbidity. For example, the impact of concurrent hypertension and diabetes on stroke mortality can be determined and monitored prospectively.

As with any surveillance system, action based on system findings is needed to complete the cycle of data collection, analysis, dissemination, and public health response. Investigation of individual case reports has not been a key feature of chronic disease surveillance, although investigation of cancer clusters often is an action of importance to community residents. Chronic disease surveillance systems can be used, for example, in monitoring potential ecologic correlations, including possible associations of high disease rates with local lifestyle features. More important, findings from chronic disease surveillance serve as an essential component in the overall planning and evaluation of chronic disease control programs. For instance, a state health department would have difficulty determining the effectiveness of a breast cancer control program without a surveillance system for mammography use, for breast cancer detection, for stage of breast cancer at time of diagnosis, and finally, for mortality.

CONTRASTS BETWEEN COMMUNICABLE
AND CHRONIC DISEASE SURVEILLANCE

Communicable disease surveillance traditionally involves identifying an illness in an individual and notifying local and state health departments, and, in some cases, the Centers for Disease Control (CDC). The intent of the system is to notify health officials and allow follow-up, if needed. The information transmitted may include personal identifiers; it may have considerable clinical detail and incorporate a specific case definition. Health officials generally build a surveillance database by accumulating reports, usually on a single disease. The system emphasizes case investigation, outbreak control, and intervention targeted toward individuals or small groups.[4]

In contrast, chronic disease surveillance currently involves the use of existing databases, which generally were not designed or collected with disease surveillance in mind. The public health response is oriented toward community intervention and control rather than individual treatment, so individual case follow-up has not been a feature, and, in fact, is often impossible because identification of individuals is not possible. Public health officials obtain information from the surveillance system by relating the elements of the various data sets to measures of interest, such as incidence, prevalence, risk, disability, and cost. Although the depth of information for a single disease is limited, perhaps including only demographic characteristics, considerable information is available for comorbid conditions and medical procedures. Diseases are identified using the *International Classification of Diseases, Ninth Revision, Clinical Modifications*, rather than specific case definitions.

The diseases monitored by many chronic disease surveillance systems may be changed as program needs and priorities change. By using ongoing data systems that include complete files for all deaths or hospitalizations in a defined population, a surveillance program can have the flexibility of choosing new surveillance endpoints to easily meet changing public health priorities The ideal chronic disease system is not oriented toward a single disease but, rather, to a broad spectrum of diseases, risk factors, and health care practices. The system emphasizes the summarization of long-term trends and patterns, the assessment of changing risks and exposures, and their analytic correlation.

DATA SOURCES FOR CHRONIC DISEASE SURVEILLANCE

For national surveillance, various data sources are available from the CDC's National Center for Health Statistics (NCHS)[5] and numerous states.[6] When used alone, any of these data systems may give only a partial picture of chronic disease burden because they usually lack unique identifiers that would allow the linkage of multiple records for one person over time. Furthermore, this lack of unique identifiers often prevents the direct linkage of related information across multiple data sets. Because no one data source gives a complete picture of disease burden, it is best to use multiple data sources.[7]

Before an existing data source is used for chronic disease surveillance, its information should be evaluated for potential usefulness in chronic disease studies.[8] Records in the data set should represent the disease of interest with some definable probability. Each record does not need verification of diagnosis, but some measure of accuracy of diagnosis for the entire data set is desirable. The data source should have a definable denominator or population base. For example, for a data set containing all hospital discharges for a single state, the state's population serves as the denominator. Individual records must be easy to manipulate to produce overall age-, race-, and sex-specific summary rates. Direct measures of epidemiologic interest, such as incidence and prevalence, may not be possible to calculate. For example, hospital data sets provide hospital discharge rates, which, while not easily converted into incidence or prevalence rates, provide a useful measure of disease burden in the community. Lastly, data collection should be ongoing to allow for continuous monitoring of disease occurrence.

Mortality Data

Vital records are an easily accessible and inexpensive source of information on disease mortality trends and geographic patterns, since virtually all deaths in the United States are recorded. National standards for the collection, processing, and coding of causes of death and other information from death certificates help to ensure that data generally are of high quality. Information on underlying and contributing causes of death from 1968 to the present are available in machine-readable form from the NCHS. Published reports include information on the underlying causes of deaths for most of this century. Selected demographic information on decedents at the county, state, and national levels also is available.[5]

Vital records alone are most useful when disease mortality trends reflect disease incidence trends, as in the case of lung cancer.[9] Vital records will not, however, reflect chronic disease incidence for conditions, such as arthritis, that do not cause or contribute to death. For surveillance of the major preventable chronic diseases, mortality data should be used along with other health outcome data sources to obtain information about morbidity in addition to mortality. Finally, for most chronic diseases, multiple-cause-of-death data are preferable to underlying-cause-of-death data, because the latter may seriously underestimate the burden of some chronic diseases; diabetes mellitus is one example.

Hospital Discharge Data

Hospital discharge data may be the only source of morbidity data for many diseases. Currently, in most hospital data systems, unique individual identifiers are not available; therefore frequency counts represent hospital discharge *events* rather than *persons* discharged from hospitals. Thus, surveillance officials may have difficulty determining initial or incident hospitalization. Despite this limitation, hospital discharge rates can serve as a useful measure of disease burden.[10] In addition, hospital discharge rates may reflect other factors, such as national health care policies and regional health care practices, access to outpatient care, and adequacy of outpatient diagnostic and treatment practices. Listed below are some major sources of hospital data.

National Hospital Discharge Survey (NHDS)

The NHDS, conducted by the NCHS, is a two-stage probability sample of approximately 200,000 hospital records collected each year from more than 400 short-stay hospitals. The NHDS is a continuous survey and, as is true for most NCHS surveys, is designed to produce accurate national and regional estimates for a wide range of diseases and for a large number of covariates. Geographic specification does not extend to the state or local levels. The NHDS also excludes Veterans Administration hospital patients, who account for about 3 percent of all reported hospitalizations. The NHDS does not include any type of unique identifying numbers on record abstracts, so multiple hospitalizations for individuals cannot be linked, and incidence rates cannot be derived.[5] In several recent reports, NHDS data have been used to estimate baseline morbidity trends for coronary heart disease,[11] cerebrovascular disease,[12] and asthma.[13, 14]

Medicare Data

The Health Care Financing Administration collects information on all hospitalizations among Medicare beneficiaries. Because Medicare covers at least 95 percent of all Americans 65 years of age and older, these data are an excellent source of information on the hospitalization experience of the elderly population.

For national surveillance of chronic diseases in persons over age 65, the Medicare hospitalization data set has several distinct advantages over the NHDS. First, Medicare records contain unique individual identifiers, thus allowing surveillance and epidemiologic studies of persons as well as hospital discharges. In addition, Medicare records contain county and ZIP codes of residence, allowing surveillance staff to calculate rates for small areas. Finally, a separate denominator file is available that allows the accurate estimation of rates for subgroups of beneficiaries.

Because they are derived from a large number of records, Medicare data can be used to generate stable rates that can be simultaneously stratified by gender, race, and age. In 1988, for example, cerebrovascular disease had the second highest crude hospitalization rate among 49 discrete conditions examined. Rates were higher for blacks in the youngest age group (65 to 74 years), but racial differences diminished with age. Little difference between the sexes was apparent.[15]

Medicare hospitalization records also contain financial information, making them useful for assessing part of the economic burden of chronic diseases in the elderly. In 1987, seven chronic diseases (diseases of the heart, malignant neoplasms, cerebrovascular disease, chronic obstructive pulmonary diseases, diabetes mellitus, atherosclerosis, and the combined category of nephritis, nephrotic syndrome, and nephrosis) accounted for 39 percent of all hospital discharges for persons aged 65 and older. Of the more than $39 billion that Medicare provided in hospital reimbursement that year, almost $17 billion (43 percent) was spent for hospitalizations in which the principal diagnosis was a major chronic disease.[16]

State-based Systems

Thirty-eight states have some form of population-based hospital discharge data system. These systems were usually established for financial monitoring and planning purposes, but increasingly state health departments are incorporating discharge data systems into their state surveillance programs. In recent years, more state hospital discharge systems have started including unique identifying numbers on record abstracts, thus allowing the linkage of multiple hospitalizations for an individual. To safeguard the confidentiality of patient information, hospital discharge data commissions usually release only linked files stripped of identifiers. At least two states, California and Maine, routinely use hospital discharge data as part of a comprehensive chronic disease surveillance system.[10, 17, 18]

Disease Registries

Surveillance, Epidemiology, and End Results (SEER) Program

The SEER program was established in 1972 by the National Cancer Institute to monitor trends in cancer incidence, survival, and mortality. Although the SEER data cover only about 11 percent of the U.S. population, they are routinely used to indirectly estimate national and state cancer incidence rates.[19] Individual SEER member registries provide nearly complete ascertainment of cancer cases within geographically defined areas, and collect extensive information on diagnosis, treatment, and survival.

State Central Cancer Registries

Thirty-nine states have some type of central cancer registry; most of these are incidence registries and thus do not collect treatment and follow-up information, as is done in the SEER program. Many of these state registries are population-based and can be used for the surveillance of most cancers. The linkage of all existing state central cancer registries could provide a national cancer surveillance system that covers about 80 percent of the U.S. population.[20]

Other Disease Registries

The registry approach offers the potential for generating very accurate data to determine incidence, prevalence, and economic burden for many chronic diseases. Registries are expensive to set up and operate, and they require close cooperation among various members of the health care community. Nonetheless, many states are exploring the use of registries for chronic diseases other than cancer, such as Alzheimer's disease and end-stage renal disease.

Surveys

Behavioral Risk Factor Surveillance System (BRFSS)

This is a CDC-organized network of state surveys designed to assess the prevalence of risk factors that contribute to unnecessary chronic disease morbidity or mortality.[21] Currently, 45 states and the District of Columbia participate in the BRFSS, covering 90 percent of the U.S. population. Risk behaviors under surveillance include smoking, alcohol use, poor diet, and physical inactivity. In addition, the system collects information on self-reports of conditions such as hypertension, and the use of preventive health services such as screening mammography and pap smears. Individual states may collect information on other health issues of special local interest. Because the data are collected primarily in telephone interviews, BRFSS underrepresents poor, minority, and homeless persons.

National Health Interview Survey (NHIS)

The NHIS, a continuous nationwide sample survey conducted annually by NCHS since 1957, uses in-person interviews to collect data from about 40,000 households and contains information on an estimated 105,000 non-institutionalized U.S. civilians. Information in the survey database includes self-reports and proxy reports of numerous acute and chronic diseases and on the use of health care services. Currently, NHIS is the primary data source for investigators who estimate national prevalence rates of major chronic diseases and analyze temporal trends in prevalence.[22] NHIS is particularly useful for researchers estimating the national prevalence of less serious conditions that do not require hospitalization, such as arthritis. Moreover, NHIS can be used to indirectly estimate state prevalence rates.[23]

National Health and Nutrition Examination Survey (NHANES)

This is a series of surveys that collects four types of data: dietary information, hematological and biochemical measurements, body measurements, and clinical assessments (medical history and physical examination). Although the surveys are not conducted continuously, and therefore are not ideal for ongoing surveillance of major chronic diseases, NHANES data can be useful as a tool for validating self-reports and proxy reports of chronic disease occurrence. Medical information included in the survey database was collected in a standardized fashion on a large representative sample of the U.S. population, thus allowing researchers to generalize findings for the nation.[6] Also available is a Hispanic NHANES, which provides information on chronic conditions in Mexican-Americans, Cuban-Americans, and Puerto Ricans.

Ambulatory Care

Information from primary or specialty care providers may be an important surveillance source for information on chronic diseases that are not so severe as to lead to hospitalization or rapid death. Large, population-based data systems for ambulatory care providers generally do not exist, although a number of large health maintenance organizations (HMOs) maintain computerized record systems. Data from these systems can provide complete health information, including both hospital care and ambulatory care, for certain sub-groups of a state population. HMO data may be particularly useful for investigators studying the natural history of selected chronic diseases.

Insurance claims data systems may be another useful source of information on ambulatory care. Currently, the Hawaii Department of Health is conducting a pilot project to determine if a statewide insurance claims data system could be used for the surveillance of both chronic and communicable diseases.[24] If the system is found to be useful, it could provide large volumes of information and a minimal lag time between physician encounter and data availability for surveillance.

REPORTING OF CHRONIC DISEASE SURVEILLANCE FINDINGS

Chronic disease surveillance findings may be used to describe an existing or emerging health problem, to assist in program evaluation, and to prompt further epidemiologic studies. The content and format for reporting the findings of chronic disease surveillance, as with other types of surveillance, are determined by the objectives of the surveillance system, its audience, and the vehicles available for dissemination. The audience for such findings is broad, including public health and medical practitioners, public health policymakers, and the general public. Such information helps medical practitioners to meet their ongoing interests in disease trends, changes in the public's knowledge of risk factors and its use of preventive services, and changes in physicians' use of diagnostic and therapeutic procedures. Epidemiologists in public health settings and in the academic community use chronic disease surveillance information to generate etiologic hypotheses, stimulate analytic studies, and develop prevention and control strategies. Chronic disease program managers and administrators use surveillance findings to help determine whether an intervention program is meeting its objectives. Finally, individual citizens find such information useful when they consider their own risk of disease and the kinds of behavioral changes they may wish to adopt.

Many vehicles are available for disseminating chronic disease surveillance findings, and the one chosen should reflect the intended audience. For the public health and medical communities, state medical journals and other professional journals reach a broad audience. State and local health department publications, such as annual reports, monthly bulletins, special individual and series reports on chronic disease, are useful for disseminating surveillance information. Such vehicles provide the greatest level of control over the presentation of results. The CDC publications useful for this purpose include the *Morbidity and Mortality Weekly Report (MMWR)* and the *CDC Surveillance Summaries*. Various professional meetings also provide a forum for sharing surveillance findings. For public health policymakers, special reports may also be advantageous. In addressing the need for public information, policymakers often distribute press releases before releasing various publications to stimulate news coverage.

As chronic disease surveillance matures, we need to determine the frequency with which surveillance findings should be reported. In contrast to frequent changes in infectious disease measures, monthly or seasonal changes in chronic disease measures are not meaningful. However, quarterly changes in mammography screening have been noted following public health interventions. Nonetheless, whether behavior changes need to be tracked every year remains a subject of debate in the public health community.

GOVERNMENT LEVELS OF RESPONSIBILITY FOR CHRONIC DISEASE SURVEILLANCE

The Institute of Medicine Report, *The Future of Public Health,* identifies the assessment of health status as one of three core functions of national, state, and local health agencies.[25] The levels of analysis involved in chronic disease surveillance vary at the different levels of government.

The federal government is responsible for establishing nationwide health objectives and priorities. To fulfill this obligation, federal officials must collect and analyze chronic disease data at the national level and provide technical assistance to help states and localities to determine their own objectives and to meet national and regional objectives.

The federal government's greatest interest is in national disease rates and the overall distribution of risks and outcomes. The emphasis is on sociodemographic differences, long- and short-term trends, and ecologic correlations. For states, the focus is on determining area-specific rates and the distribution of rates across the state, identifying high risk groups, targeting programs, and health planning. For local health departments, surveillance information is used for defining the resources needed to control programs.

SUMMARY

Chronic disease surveillance, a relatively new component of public health practice, differs significantly from the surveillance of infectious diseases. A number of data sets are used, each with specific strengths and limitations. The goals of chronic disease surveillance differ at national, state, and local levels. The pace of demographic change and the growing societal burden of chronic diseases will demand attention and, one would hope, will accelerate the development of better chronic disease surveillance systems.

ACKNOWLEDGMENTS

We would like to thank Richard B. Rothenberg, M.D., and the staff of the CDC's Chronic Disease Surveillance Branch, for their contributions to this chapter.

Notes
1. Thacker, S. B. and R. L. Berkelman. 1988. Public health surveillance in the United States. *Epidemiol Rev* 10:164–190.
2. Centers for Disease Control. 1988. Changes in premature mortality: United States, 1979–1986. *MMWR* 37:47–48.
3. Rothenberg, R. B., and J. P. Koplan. 1990. Chronic disease in the 1990s. *Ann Rev Public Health* 11:267–296.

4. Langmuir, A. D. 1963. The surveillance of communicable diseases of national importance. *NEJM* 268:182–192.
5. Kovar, M. G. 1989. Data systems of the National Center for Health Statistics. *Vital Health Stat* 1:2223.
6. Centers for Disease Control. 1987. Survey of chronic disease activities in state and territorial health agencies. *MMWR* 36:565–568.
7. Lentzner, H. R., J. M. Mendlein, L. Graham, G. A. Kaplan, W. Perry, and W. Wright. Development of state chronic disease surveillance systems. In: *Challenges for Public Health Statistics in the 1990s*, 181–186. Washington, D.C.: National Center for Health Statistics, 1989.
8. Centers for Disease Control. 1988. *Guidelines for Evaluating Surveillance Systems: 1988*. Atlanta, Ga.: CDC.
9. Centers for Disease Control. 1990. Trends in lung cancer incidence and mortality: United States, 1980–1987. *MMWR* 39:875, 881–883.
10. Centers for Disease Control. 1989. Smoking-attributable mortality, morbidity, and economic costs: California, 1985. *MMWR* 38:272–275.
11. Centers for Disease Control. 1989. Hospital discharge rates for ischemic heart disease, 1970–1986. *MMWR* 38:275–284.
12. Centers for Disease Control. 1989. Hospital discharge rates for cerebrovascular disease, 1970–1986. *MMWR* 38:194–210.
13. Centers for Disease Control. 1990. Asthma: United States, 1980–1987. *MMWR* 39:493–497.
14. Evans, R., III, D. I. Mullally, R. W. Wilson et al. 1987. National trends in the morbidity and mortality of asthma in the U.S.: prevalence, hospitalization, and death from asthma over two decades, 1965–1984. *Chest* 91(suppl): 65S–74S.
15. May, D. S., J. J. Kelly, J. M. Mendlein, and P. L. Garbe. 1991. Surveillance of major causes of hospitalization among the elderly, 1988. In: CDC surveillance summaries, April 1991. *MMWR* 40(No. SS-1):7–21.
16. Centers for Disease Control. 1990. Hospitalizations for the leading causes of death among the elderly: United States, 1987. *MMWR* 39:777–779, 785.
17. California Department of Health Services. 1991. Ischemic heart disease, hypertension, and cerebrovascular disease deaths and hospitalizations: California, 1983–1987. Berkeley, Ca.: CDHS.
18. Maine Department of Human Services and Maine Health Care Finance Commission. 1989. *Maine Chronic and Sentinel Disease Surveillance Project: 1984–1986 Report*. Augusta, Maine: MDHS and MHCFC.
19. National Cancer Institute. 1981. *Surveillance, Epidemiology, and End Results: Incidence and Mortality Data, 1973–1977*, 1–9. Washington, D.C.: National Institutes of Health, Department of Health and Human Services, NIH pub. no. 81-2330.
20. Donald Austin, M.D. Personal communication, 1990.
21. Remington, P. L., M. Y. Smith, D. F. Williamson, R. F. Anda, E. M. Gentry, and G. C. Hogelin. 1988. Design, characteristics, and usefulness of state-based behavioral risk factor surveillance: 1981–1987. *Public Health Rep* 103:366–376.

22. National Center for Health Statistics. 1977. Washington, D.C.: U.S. Government Printing Office pub. no. 60713, 186–273.
23. Centers for Disease Control. 1990. Prevalence of arthritic conditions: United States. *MMWR* 39:99–102.
24. Robert Worth, M.D., Ph.D. Personal communication, March 1991.
25. Institute of Medicine. 1988. *The Future of Public Health,* 7–10. Washington, D.C.: National Academy Press.

11

Injury Surveillance

Philip L. Graitcer

Since the publication of *Injury in America*[1] in 1985, increased public health interest has been directed toward reducing and preventing injuries. While much of this attention has resulted in increased support for basic and operational research in acute care, biomechanics, and rehabilitation, significant resources also have been devoted to the development of public health injury prevention programs. As part of these prevention programs, public health surveillance is being used to quantify the health and financial burdens of injuries on the population, to identify possible risk factors and determinants associated with injuries, and to evaluate existing injury prevention programs. Injury surveillance also can be used to make important contributions to other phases of injury control, such as acute care, treatment, and rehabilitation. This chapter will review some of these injury surveillance activities, compare and contrast injury and communicable disease surveillance, discuss commonly used sources of injury surveillance data, and describe what minimum data variables should be collected in an injury surveillance system. In addition, I will describe three injury surveillance systems that are representative of systems being developed by public health agencies.

THE IMPACT OF INJURIES

Each year, nearly one in every four Americans is injured. In 1986 alone, about 57 million persons were injured, according to U.S. health survey data. Falls, the single most frequent cause of injury, account for about one-fifth of all injuries.[2] Injury remains the number one cause of death for persons between 1 and 44 years of age, and it is the fourth leading cause

142

of death overall. In 1987, almost 150,000 Americans died as a result of injuries. About one-third of all fatal injuries occur in motor vehicle crashes, and another third result from acts of violence, such as suicide (60 percent of all violent deaths) and homicide.[2] Furthermore, each year injuries send millions of Americans to the hospital. In 1985, about 2.3 million persons were hospitalized for injuries.[2] One-third of these hospitalizations were the result of falls. In addition, injuries place a multibillion-dollar burden on the U.S. economy in terms of direct costs and the cost of lost or reduced productivity. In 1987, that burden was estimated to total at least $180 billion.[2]

INJURY SURVEILLANCE
AND COMMUNICABLE
DISEASE SURVEILLANCE

Only recently have injury surveillance activities been developed as part of injury control programs. Most of these injury surveillance activities are based on principles that have been developed and refined for communicable disease surveillance.[4] Injury surveillance and communicable disease surveillance are conducted for the same general purposes: to provide a quantitative estimate of morbidity and mortality, to detect clusters, to stimulate epidemiologic research, and to help evaluate the effectiveness of interventions. Similarities and differences in the nature of communicable diseases and injuries, however, require us to reconsider traditional methods when conducting injury surveillance.

Case Definition

In communicable disease surveillance, a disease is identified by clinical signs, symptoms, or laboratory measures. For example, the surveillance case definition for viral hepatitis is "an illness characterized by discrete onset of jaundice and/or elevated serum aminotransferase levels. Viral hepatitis cases are further subdivided based on . . . serologic tests."[5] The word "injury" can have several meanings, depending on whether it is being used in clinical, research, or epidemiological settings. For instance, an injury could be defined as the *outcome* of an adverse event (broken leg, crushed chest). Alternatively, an injury could be the *event* leading to an adverse event, such as a fall or a motorcycle crash. Because we are interested in the epidemiological aspects of injuries, we will use the second definition; that is, an event that leads to trauma. Our definition should be further narrowed according to our particular research or public health objectives. For instance, we can define an injury on the basis of the level of medical care given (hospitalization, emergency room visit, or physician's office visit), the injury outcome (complete recovery, permanent or temporary paralysis, death), the place where it occurred (daycare center, home), the type of activity that occurred (sports and leisure, occupational), or the event itself (a fall from a ladder, a fall down stairs, or a fall from a motorcycle). Furthermore, risk factors (such as alcohol or drug use), the use of prevention devices (seat belts, smoke detectors), and intentionality (homicide, assault) are used to qualify an injury case definition.

The selection of a case definition for injury surveillance depends ultimately on the objectives for conducting surveillance. If the purpose of surveillance is to determine the occurrence of an injury in a community, then the case definition should be chosen to include all levels of severity or outcome, and data on all cases of that injury should be collected. To quantify the morbidity and mortality impact of fall injuries in the elderly, public health officials in Miami Beach, Florida, collected surveillance data on all fall injuries for persons over 65 years of age, including those falls that resulted in death, hospitalization, or an outpatient visit.[6] Similarly, to aid in the development of a public health program to prevent serious burn injuries, the Oklahoma Department of Health collected surveillance data from all burn injuries that resulted in death or admission to a hospital burn unit.[7]

Data Sources

Injury surveillance is often conducted by using many of the data sources commonly used for communicable disease surveillance, such as physician and hospital reports, medical examiners' records, and household surveys. Frequently, supplemental, less commonly used sources of data are used. These data are generally collected for purposes other than for injury surveillance and consequently may need additional data variables to be useful for surveillance. Examples of data sources used for the surveillance of injury severity, outcome, or intent include fire and public safety reports,[8] the Uniform Crime Reports of the Federal Bureau of Investigation (FBI),[9] the Fatal Accident Reporting System (FARS),[10] U.S. Coast Guard Boat Accident Reporting System,[11] the National Spinal Cord Injury Network,[12] and the National Athletic Injury/Illness Reporting System (NAIRS).[13]

Multiple sources of data frequently are needed to identify all cases that result from a particular injury. In a study of fatalities in all-terrain vehicles in Alaska, data from vital records, public safety records, medical examiner's reports, a news clipping service, and the Consumer Product Safety

Commission were used to document all the fatal cases.[14] None of these data sources alone could be used to identify all fatal all-terrain vehicle injuries.

Etiology

Injuries usually have a multifactorial etiology, which makes the identification of potential risk factors difficult. For example, to identify possible risk factors associated with motor vehicle crashes, data on the road conditions, vehicles, and use of personal protective devices such as seat belts should be collected. Similarly, to determine some of the risk factors that result in house fire–associated burns, information is needed about building construction, fire department response, and the presence or absence of smoke detectors. To describe the complex interaction of risk factors involved in injury causation and to develop targeted interventions, it may be necessary to supplement surveillance data with information obtained from detailed epidemiologic studies, such as case control studies.

Clustering

Analyses of time clusters for the identification of injury outbreaks are often not satisfactory for conducting injury surveillance. Although injuries occur in clusters—such as when several persons die in airplane crashes, suicide clusters,[15] or from the use of unsafe products such as an all-terrain vehicle[14]—more commonly, injury deaths occur in isolation or in pairs. Overall, although about 390 injury fatalities occur each day in the United States, their appearance is often spread out over a large geographic area, rendering traditional surveillance techniques such as voluntary physician or sentinel reporting ineffective.

SOURCES OF INJURY SURVEILLANCE DATA

Injury surveillance systems often use data sources that have been developed for other purposes. For example, hospital trauma registries are used primarily to aid in the assessment of quality of patient care and traditionally have included little information on the injury event. Recently, however, they are being expanded to include information on the cause of the injury-producing event.[16] Because data sources for injury surveillance often have been collected for purposes other than prevention, they may fail to include critical facts, be imprecise, or be out of date, thus limiting their value for injury surveillance.[17] Efforts are underway to use some of these data sources for public health surveillance by either expanding the data sets or by linking them with other data sources that could contain additional epidemiological data.[4]

The most readily available data sources are compiled nationally. These sources are useful for obtaining information on the overall impact or distribution of an injury. Regional and local sources specific to a community, however, should be used for the planning and evaluation of that community's programs. In this section, I will describe commonly used national data sources and suggest sources that could be used on a community level.

Mortality Data

Several sources of data, generally available throughout the United States, are commonly used to conduct surveillance for fatal injuries: death certificates, medical examiner reports, the FBI's Supplemental Homicide Reports, and FARS. Of these sources, death certificates are the most frequently used. All deaths in the United States are recorded by state and vital statistics jurisdictions on death certificates using a standardized protocol. The injury that started the sequence of events leading to death is coded as the underlying cause of death. The cause is coded according to the current version of the International Classification of Diseases (ICD) Supplemental Classification of External Cause of Death (or E-code), which describes the external cause of injury.[18] Using vital statistics data, coded with the external cause of injury, epidemiologic studies and ongoing surveillance have been conducted.[19]

Medical examiner's and coroner's reports provide additional, and sometimes detailed, sources of injury mortality data for some injury deaths. In most states, medical examiners or coroners are required to investigate and determine the cause of any sudden or unexpected death. The medical examiner's report contains these investigations plus additional medical information such as toxicological and autopsy data. Although medical examiner's reports are useful for the surveillance of injury fatalities and are often available in a timely manner, they are rarely computerized, they are not consistent from jurisdiction to jurisdiction, and, as with death certificates, they may not contain critical epidemiological information, such as whether seat belts were used or whether or not the fatality was occupationally related.[20] Collaborative efforts with members of the National Association of Medical Examiners and the Centers for Disease Control are underway to address these deficiencies.[21]

State public safety or highway departments investigate fatal motor vehicle crashes that occur on public highways. With the support of the National Highway Traffic Safety Administration (NHTSA), these investigations are coded, analyzed, and compiled into a national database, the Fatal Accident Reporting System (FARS).[10] State and regional officials may obtain printed tabulations and computer tapes of the FARS data from NHTSA. The FARS data, however, lack specific medical information about the decedents in these crashes; specifically, the causes of deaths, medical diagnoses, and blood alcohol levels of all drivers and passengers. Reports are limited to deaths that occurred within 30 days of the motor vehicle crash. To obtain more medical details about persons fatally injured in motor vehicle crashes, a pilot test is being conducted that links the FARS data to national death certificate data.[22]

The Supplementary Homicide Report, part of the FBI's Uniform Crime Report, contains information on the age, race, and sex of the victim and offender, the relationship of the offender to the victim, and information on the crime circumstances. These reports are completed by local, county, and state law enforcement agencies and are compiled by the FBI. These data are complete for about 90 to 95 percent of the total murder and nonnegligent manslaughter cases.[23]

Other data sources, such as the National Fire Incident Reporting System[8] and the U.S. Coast Guard database of commercial vessel casualties,[11] need to be further evaluated to determine their usefulness for injury surveillance, especially at the state and local levels. State agencies such as departments of agriculture, natural resources, and labor often collect data on fatalities and injury events occurring in their administrative jurisdictions. These data sources can be useful surveillance data sources in selected community injury prevention programs.

Morbidity Data

Several periodic national surveys collect data that are potentially useful for injury morbidity surveillance. The National Center for Health Statistics (NCHS) conducts the National Health Interview Survey (NHIS).[24] This door-to-door national survey is designed to represent the civilian, noninstitutional U.S. population. Information on injury is collected by asking the respondent whether or not he or she has had a traumatic injury within the past 14 days that restricted activity or required medical attention. NHIS data are not routinely given E-codes, and information on the cause of injury is limited. Intentionality of the injury cannot be determined from the survey. Also, because a relatively small number of people are actually surveyed for most injuries, except motor vehicle injuries, the actual number of case reports is too small to reliably estimate national incidence.

Two other surveys conducted by NCHS, the National Hospital Discharge Survey (NHDS)[25] and the National Ambulatory Medical Care Survey (MAMCS),[25] collect data on injury visits to hospitals and office-based physicians that are useful for injury surveillance. Although neither of these surveys contains records that are routinely given E-codes or that contain supplemental information on the cause or intentionality of the injury, anticipated modifications in hospital discharge coding requirements will increase the availability of records that include cause of injury data.

The Consumer Product Safety Commission (CPSC) collects injury data from several sources and is used to identify injuries related to the use of consumer products. These sources include injury reports from medical examiners, a news clipping service, consumer complaints, and hospital emergency department visits that result in medical treatment. The hospital emergency department source, known as the National Electronic Injury Surveillance System (NEISS),[26] uses a nationally representative sample of 64 hospital emergency departments to gather information on injuries seen in these departments. Data on injuries not related to consumer products or injuries caused by products not under the CPSC's jurisdiction (such as firearms and motor vehicles) are not collected. Information on intentionality is not collected. A second level of the NEISS surveillance involves case investigations designed to collect detailed information on injuries related to certain products. It is through this combination of emergency room surveillance and case investigation that the CPSC has been able to identify potentially hazardous consumer products such as all-terrain vehicles and lawn darts.

The Department of Justice's National Crime Survey collects data on morbidity that is associated with interpersonal violence.[9]

Presently, we lack adequate national health data sources that accurately measure the morbid impact of injuries. This is primarily because of the absence of etiologic information on medical reports of nonfatal injury.[27] Since approximately 99 percent of injuries are not fatal, this gap in injury surveillance data is particularly serious.[28] Aggregated hospital data are a prime source of information on nonfatal injuries. If the cause of an injury was routinely obtained as part of the patient history and if the hospital discharge summary was classified by E-codes discharge data would be extremely useful for surveillance.

Data from a hospital discharge data (HDD) system contains a standard set of information about all patients discharged from acute care hospitals. Twenty-eight states presently have HDD systems or regulations requiring them to develop an HDD system.[29] Only six states—California, Michigan, New York, Rhode Island, Vermont, and Washington—require that cause-of-injury E-codes be included in the HDD system. Without E-codes, however, HDD are less useful for injury surveillance. HDD do not distinguish between initial hospital admissions and discharges for an injury and subsequent hospitalizations for treatment of the same injury. As a result, the number of injury events may be overestimated in the hospital discharge database. Additionally, these data are often not compiled until 2 to 4 years after the discharge, making them less valuable for the detection of clusters of injury problems.

Some special hospital systems, most notably the U.S. Public Health Service's Indian Health Service hospital systems, code hospital discharge data with cause-of-injury codes. As a result, these data sets can be used for public health surveillance.[30]

Trauma registries are a potential source for local injury surveillance data. Complete patient data, including information on the nature of the injury, emergency room or inpatient hospital course, as well as discharge data on outcome and medical costs, are usually available on trauma registries. By linking trauma registry data to other records that contain additional nonmedical information on the injury event or risk factors, these registries can provide the local surveillance data needed to target and evaluate certain injury interventions. One major limitation of using trauma registry data for injury surveillance is a lack of representativeness. Trauma registry data are representative only of those persons injured severely enough to be taken to the trauma center. Deaths that occur at the scene of the event, injuries not requiring trauma system care, and injuries treated at other trauma centers are not included in the database. Also, a trauma registry may not contain information for all types of injuries, such as near-drownings. Trauma data have, however, proved useful. In Texas, data from a trauma center were used to describe differences in survival rates, injuries, and medical care costs between helmeted and unhelmeted motorcycle operators. Although information on motorcycle helmet usage was not available in the trauma registry database, the trauma record was linked to the Texas Department of Public Safety officer's report of the motorcycle crash.[31]

Special registries, such as those developed for head and spinal cord injuries, burns, and poisonings have been established in several states. The main purpose of these registries is to maintain a case listing of injured persons that can aid in providing appropriate rehabilitative, vocational, and financial assistance, or to evaluate the quality of medical care in specialized health systems. By including information on the cause of injury, these registries also can be used for surveillance and for other epidemiologic studies of injuries, such as case-control studies of specific risk factors and interventions.[32]

Emergency department medical records or log sheets are frequently proposed as data sources for local injury surveillance. Hospital and freestanding emergency departments receive a large number of injury cases, and these cases may include a wide range of injuries, both by type and severity. Unlike the NEISS emergency department records that are collected by specially trained records administrators in a representative sample of hospitals, data collected from emergency department records have several limitations when used for injury surveillance. Case records or log sheets rarely include information on the cause or severity of injuries. Emergency department records may not be computerized, and there are frequently large numbers of cases at all levels of severity.[33] As a result, extensive personnel and financial resources are often required for the collection and analysis of injury surveillance data from emergency departments. A sampling of these records could reduce the resource burden needed for data collection and analysis. The primary limitation in using emergency department data for injury surveillance is its lack of representativeness. Deaths at the scene, trauma registry cases, and injuries either treated at other hospitals or not treated do not appear in the database. Because of their lack of representativeness, lack of computerization, and frequent need for extensive resources to collect and analyze the surveillance data, emergency department records are generally considered less satisfactory as a primary source for injury surveillance in a community.

Additional sources of morbidity data include police and fire reports, emergency medical service "trip" reports, highway police motor vehicle accident reports, and industrial and day-care center medical logs. The usefulness and limitations of using these data sources for injury surveillance have not been evaluated.

DATA VARIABLES FOR
INJURY SURVEILLANCE

Although the choice of data variables for injury surveillance depends on the purposes for conducting the surveillance and the injury event under investigation, certain variables should always be included in injury surveillance (see Table 11-1). This minimum data set is designed to provide basic epidemiologic elements of person, place, and time, along with information about the nature, cause, and outcome of the injury. Before other variables are added to the minimum data set, consideration should be given to the additional resources needed to collect these variables, and whether they are useful in conducting research and prevention programs.

INJURY SURVEILLANCE SYSTEMS

Injury surveillance systems often require that data from several sources be obtained, linked, and analyzed to establish comprehensive data rec-

TABLE 11-1   Minimum Data Set for Injury Surveillance

Person	Give age, sex, race, and place of residence of the person injured. If this is an intentional injury, the same variables on the perpetrator would also be useful.
Location	Specify place where the injury occurred, such as school, home, work, ballfield.
Time	List day and time when the injury occurred.
Nature of Injury	Identify part(s) of body injured, such as fractured left arm.
Cause of Injury	Describe how and why the injury occurred. If possible, use an E-code.
Diagnosis	Specify the diagnosis using N-codes.
Outcome	Specify whether treated and released, hospitalized, temporary or permanent loss of function, death.
Other Factors	Indicate, for example, seat belt/motorcycle helmet use; alcohol or drug use.

ords.[12] By using more than one data source, a surveillance system's overall usefulness can be improved; however, the cost of conducting surveillance and operating the system may be higher and data collection in the system may be less acceptable to the personnel collecting and analyzing data. This section discusses several surveillance systems that have been implemented, each of which uses a different methodology and different sources of data.

Reportable Injuries: Oklahoma Spinal Cord Surveillance

In 1987, the Oklahoma Department of Health established surveillance for traumatic spinal cord injuries (SCI). The ultimate goal of this surveillance was to develop an SCI prevention program. It was necessary to obtain data from all cases of SCI in the state; however, neither a spinal cord injury registry nor a hospital discharge data system existed. SCI was designated by the health commissioner as a reportable health condition. This meant that physicians and hospitals were required to submit information on SCI to the health department. All hospitals, neurologists, and neurosurgeons in the state were contacted and made aware of the reporting requirements and the surveillance case definition for SCI. They were also given a specially designed data collection form. Additionally, the medical examiner's office was asked to provide case reports on all fatal injuries that would have met the case definition for an SCI. Staff of the Department of Health periodically called and visited the hospitals and physicians to stimulate reporting of spinal cord injury data. Periodic analyses of the data were completed by the Health Department and were disseminated to health practitioners throughout the state. One important finding during the first year of surveillance was the higher incidence of spinal cord injuries with pick-up truck crashes compared with other types of motor vehicle crashes. A follow-up study is being conducted to learn more about SCI risk factors related to pick-up truck crashes.[34]

Active Surveillance Using Special Forms: the National Boy Scout Jamboree and the Peace Corps

Quadrennially, the national Boy Scout Jamboree is held at an Army training camp in Virginia. A surveillance system is established by the U.S. Public Health Service to characterize severe injuries that may occur in youths attending this summer camp and to act as an early warning system that will identify potentially hazardous events and activities. In each camp subsector, a nurse completes a standard injury report form before referring the scout to the hospital. This form includes basic demographic data as well as information on the site and type of activity, time of the injury, and nature of the injury. The survey forms are collected daily and their accuracy is verified. In addition, log books from the hospital are reviewed to determine completeness of survey coverage. Significant findings from the surveillance system are reviewed daily at staff meetings with Boy Scout personnel, and situations or activities associated with injuries are investigated and, if necessary, modified to correct the existing hazard. In 1985, this sytem identified two activities, the BMX bike course and the bucking bronco, associated with substantially higher numbers of injuries than other activities. Environmental modifications were made to these events and further injuries to the scouts were prevented.[35]

A similar, single-purpose surveillance system for Peace Corps volunteers serving abroad was recently established. This system used a specially designed injury report form that was completed by the Peace Corps medical officer and the volunteer following an injury. The system identified loss of control of motorcycles as the cause of more than 50 percent of all injuries. Intensified motorcycle safety training and stricter enforcement of safety regulations for Peace Corps volunteers were implemented to reduce these injuries.[36]

Surveillance Using Emergency Department Records: the Oregon Injury Registry

In 1985, the Oregon Division of Health established a pilot injury registry system designed to provide information on the statewide distribution of injuries to aid in planning for a regionalized system of trauma care and to help hospitals meet requirements for accreditation by providing them with patient visit information. Initially, the system was designed to cover all hospitals in six counties. Each hospital was given computer programs, training, and assistance in establishing an emergency department patient registry database. The database was constructed to provide information on patient demographics, treatment, and disposition. In addition, information on the cause of injury was collected both as an E-code and as a narrative description of the injury event. Data were entered on each injury patient admitted to the hospital. Hospitals had the capability to analyze the data locally, and each month they shared a diskette containing the patient data with the Division of Health. Cases of fatal injury were obtained from the Oregon Medical Examiner, and further analyses were conducted by the Division of Health. These data have been used to assist the health department in targeting childhood injury programs and in helping community groups to develop head injury prevention programs.[37] The system is being expanded to include all hospitals in the state by 1991.[38]

CONCLUSIONS

Several basic principles should be considered in designing an injury surveillance system. First, the design depends on the purpose of surveillance. The case definition, the frequency of data collection and analysis, and the data sources selected depend on the objective for conducting surveillance. For example, a surveillance system for determining the distribution of SCI in a community may have a different case definition and different data sources than one designed to measure the effectiveness of an intervention to reduce SCI resulting from motor vechicle crashes. Second, various data sources can be used for injury surveillance. Important considerations in selecting a data source are the availability of cause of injury information, the representativeness of the data, and the ability to link the data source with other potentially useful data sources. Convenience in collecting and analyzing the data (such as having data in an electronic, rather than a paper, format) should also be a consideration. Existing data sources such as registries for burns, trauma, head and spinal injuries, and hospital discharge data summaries are potentially useful sources for collecting information on serious injuries. Third, injury surveillance should not be confused with case investigation. Although an injury surveillance system can be useful in the identification of cases of an injury, it is not the most efficient method to determine which risk factors cause injury. An epidemiologic study, such as a case-control study using data initially gained from a population-based surveillance system, is more appropriate to identify risk factors. Fourth, a minimal data set should be used for injury surveillance. Often in a surveillance system there is a tendency to collect too much data on too many variables. This increases cost, decreases acceptability, and unreasonably raises expectations regarding the usefulness of the surveillance system. Surveillance should be used to drive public health programs, not to determine risk factors. Lastly, local data should be used for injury surveillance. Although national surveillance is useful in the determination of the impact of injury, local sources of data must be used for targeting and evaluating the prevention program.

Notes

1. Committee on Trauma Research, National Research Council, Institute of Medicine. 1985. *Injury in America: A Continuing Public Health Problem.* Washington, D.C.: National Academy Press.
2. Baker, S. P., B. O'Neil, and R. S. Karpf. 1984. *The Injury Fact Book.* Lexington, Mass.: Lexington Books, D.C. Heath and Company.
3. Rice, D. P., E. J. MacKenzie, and Associates. 1989. *Cost of injury in the United States: A report to Congress.* San Francisco, Calif.: Institute for Health and Aging, University of California and Injury Prevention Center, Johns Hopkins University.
4. Thacker, S. B., and R. L. Berkelman. 1988. Public health surveillance in the United States. *Epidemiol Rev* 10:164–190.
5. Centers for Disease Control and the Council of State and Territorial Epidemiologists. 1989. *Case Definitions for Surveillance of Notifiable Disease.* Atlanta, Ga.: CDC.
6. DeVito, C. A., D. A. Lambert, R. W. Sattin et al. 1988. Epidemiology of fall injuries among the elderly, Dade County, Florida, 1985–1986. *J Am Geriatr Soc* 36:1029–1035.
7. Makintubee, S. 1989. Personal communication.
8. Federal Emergency Management Agency, United States Fire Administration. 1987. *Fire in the United States (1983).* 6th ed. Washington, DC: FEMA, U.S. Fire Administration, U.S. Government Printing Office (FEMA pub. no. 772-629/60498).
9. U.S. Department of Justice. *Crime in the United States, 1986.* Washington, D.C.: U.S. Department of Justice, 1987.
10. National Highway Traffic Safety Administration (NHTSA). 1981. *Fatal Accident Reporting System (FARS): User's Guide.* Washington, D.C.: NHTSA.
11. U.S. Coast Guard. 1984. *Coding Instructions for the Automated File of Commercial Vessel Casualties.* Washington, D.C.: U.S. Coast Guard.
12. Stover, S. L., and P. R. Fine, eds. 1986. *Spinal Cord Injury: The Facts and Figures.* Birmingham, Ala.: University of Alabama.
13. Clarke, K. S. 1976. Premises and pitfalls of athletic injury surveillance. *J Sport Med* 3:292–295.
14. Smith, S. M., and J. P. Middaugh. 1989. An assessment of potential injury surveillance data sources in Alaska using an emerging problem: all-terrain vehicle-associated injuries. *Public Health Rep* 104:493–498.

15. O'Carroll, P. W., J. A. Mercy, and J. A. Steward. 1988. CDC Recommendations for a community plan for the prevention and containment of suicide clusters. *MMWR* 37(suppl. no. S-6):1–12.
16. Pollock, D. A., and P. W. McClain. 1989. Trauma registries: current status and future prospects. *JAMA* 262:2280–2283.
17. Graitcer, P. L. 1987. Development of state and local injury surveillance systems. *J Safety Res* 18:191–198.
18. Health Care Financing Administration. 1980. *International Classification of Diseases*. 9th rev. ed. Washington, D.C.: U.S. Government Printing Office (DHHS pub. no. 80-1260).
19. Sosin, D. N., J. J. Sacks, and S. M. Smith. 1989. Head injury–associated deaths in the United States from 1979–1986. *JAMA* 262:2251–2255.
20. Conroy, C., and J. C. Russell. In press. Medical examiner/coroner records: uses and limitations in occupational injury epidemiologic research. *J Forensic Sci*.
21. Centers for Disease Control. 1989. Death investigation: United States, 1987. *MMWR* 38:1–4.
22. Fell, J. 1988. Personal communication.
23. Rosenberg, M. L., and J. A. Mercy. 1985. *Homicide and assaultive violence*. Background paper prepared for the Surgeon General's Conference on Violence as a Public Health Problem.
24. National Center for Health Statistics. 1985. *National Health Interview Survey: Design, 1973–84; Procedures, 1975–83*. Washington, D.C.: NCHS. Vital and Health Statistics, Series 1, Number 18.
25. National Center for Health Statistics. 1981. *Data Systems of the National Center for Health Statistics*. Washington, D.C.: NCHS. Vital and Health Statistics, Series 1, Number 16.
26. Consumer Product Safety Commission. 1984. National Electronic Injury Surveillance System (NEISS). *NEISS Data Highlights* 8:1.
27. Sniezek, J. E., F. J. Finklea, and P. L. Graitcer. 1989. Injury coding and hospital discharge data. *JAMA* 269:2270–2272.
28. Gallagher, S. S., K. Finison, B. Guyer, and S. Goodenough. 1984. The incidence of injuries among 87,000 Massachusetts children and adolescents: results of the 1980–81 Statewide Childhood Injury Prevention Program surveillance system. *Am J Public Health* 74:1340–1347.
29. *NAHDO Resource Manual*. 1988. Washington, D.C.: The National Association of Health Data Organizations.
30. Smith, S. M., B. K. Molloy, H. S. Winick, and P. L. Graitcer. In press. An epidemiologic analysis of injuries at three IHS service units. *J Environ Health*.
31. Lloyd, L. E., and P. L. Graitcer. 1989. The potential for using a trauma registry for injury surveillance and prevention. *Am J Prev Med* 5:34–37.
32. Goldberg, J., H. M. Gelfand, and P. S. Levy. 1980. Registry evaluation methods: a review and case study. *Epidemiol Rev* 2:210–220.
33. National Committee for Injury Prevention and Control. 1989. Injury prevention: meeting the challenge. *Am J Prev Med* 5(suppl):40.

34. Oklahoma State Department of Health. 1989. *Traumatic Spinal Cord Injuries Resulting from Motor Vehicle Crashes.* Internal report, January 20.
35. Wetterhall, S. F., and R. J. Waxweiler. 1988. Injury surveillance at the 1985 national Boy Scout Jamboree. *Am J Sports Med* 16:534–538.
36. Graitcer, P. L., K. L. Bernard, and T. Van Der Vlugt. 1989. Injuries in Peace Corps volunteers. *Travel Med Int* 7:153–156.
37. Oregon Division of Health. 1989. *Annual Report: Oregon Injury Registry 1987.* Portland, Oreg.: Oregon Department of Health.
38. Gordon, J. 1990. Personal communication.

12

Surveillance of Birth Defects

Michele C. Lynberg and Larry D. Edmonds

INTRODUCTION

Birth defects surveillance methodology, which has been developed during the last 25 years, continues to provide a good model for the surveillance of developmental disabilities and other chronic childhood diseases. In this chapter, we examine the objectives, attributes, and components of an ideal birth defects surveillance program. We also describe several state, national, and international birth defects surveillance systems, outline the limitations of birth defects surveillance systems, and finally, suggest ways to make birth defects surveillance more uniform.

PUBLIC HEALTH IMPORTANCE OF BIRTH DEFECTS

Birth defects are the leading cause of infant mortality in the United States, accounting for more than 21 percent of all infant deaths in 1986.[1] In addition, birth defects are the fifth leading cause of years of potential life lost[2] and contribute substantially to childhood morbidity and long-term disability. Major birth defects are diagnosed in 3 to 4 percent of infants in their first year of life. Of the approximately 100,000 to 150,000 infants born with a major birth defect each year,[3] approximately 6,000 die during their first 28 days of life, and another 2,000 die before reaching their first birthday, leaving 92,000 to 142,000 living children affected to various degrees.[4] Children with birth defects account for approximately 25 to 30 percent of pediatric admissions; total costs for care of children with birth defects exceed $1.4 billion annually.[5, 6] Using reported age-specific survival rates and age-specific medical-care costs, officials at the Centers for

Disease Control (CDC) estimate that $90 million (based on 1985 dollar equivalents) were spent on medical care by 1990 for 12,000 surviving infants born with spina bifida since 1980.[7]

DEFINITION AND CLASSIFICATION OF BIRTH DEFECTS

Definition

A birth defect is a structural abnormality present at birth; most, but not all, are included within the range 740.0 to 759.9 of the *International Classification of Diseases, Ninth Revision* (ICD-9).[8] Conditions within this category include a heterogeneous group of outcomes with differing morphogenesis, including (1) malformations, which involve poor tissue formation; (2) deformations, which involve unusual forces on normal tissue; and (3) disruptions, which involve the breakdown of normal tissue.

Classification

Most birth defects occur as isolated defects. In about 20 to 30 percent of affected infants, however, multiple defects are involved. Much work is being done to classify infants with multiple birth defects according to biologically meaningful categories that would be useful in identifying etiologic and pathogenetic mechanisms.[9] Some multiple birth defects are due to sequences (e.g., oligohydramnios, arthrogryposis), whereas others are due to recognized syndromes (e.g., chromosomal abnormalities, known teratogens), but the vast majority have no identified underlying pathogenetic or etiologic mechanisms. These multiple birth defects of unknown causes are referred to as associations (e.g., VATER: vertebral anomalies, anal atresia, T-E fistula, renal anomaly; MURCS: Muellerian duct, renal and cervical vertebral defects).

Birth defects can also be classified as major or minor; major birth defects are those that affect survival, require substantial medical care, or result in marked physiological or psychological impairment.[10]

OBJECTIVES OF BIRTH DEFECTS SURVEILLANCE

Historical Objectives

Widespread interest in birth defects surveillance was generated following the epidemic of limb reduction deformities in the early 1960s associated with the prenatal use of thalidomide. Few specific causes of birth defects were known, and the epidemiologic patterns of several malformations suggested that unidentified teratogens were important in the etiology of major congenital malformations. Interest in birth defects surveillance has continued to grow, with programs currently monitoring outcomes in several states, as well as nationally and internationally.[11, 12]

Current Objectives

In addition to being used to search for increases in the incidence of specific malformations—increases that could reflect the introduction of new teratogens or increased exposure to old ones—surveillance systems for birth defects have several other functions. They can be used to develop baseline data, provide timely rates, and identify geographic areas of concern for cluster investigations. Surveillance systems also provide the basis for both ecologic investigations and follow-up studies. By monitoring national and local birth defects rates, investigators can correlate changing trends with changes in cultural, social, and environmental factors. From a public health perspective, birth defects surveillance is important because some causes are entirely preventable. These include fetal alcohol syndrome,[13] congenital rubella,[14] and isotretinoin (Accutane)* embryopathy.[15]

Birth defects surveillance systems are also useful in the identification of infants and children with birth defects. These case registries can be used for etiologic investigations, studies of economic impact, and follow-up studies in which the long-term effects of birth defects, including the development of cancer,[16] and survival rates, are assessed.[17] Registries developed from birth defects surveillance systems are also useful in testing hypotheses and in conducting descriptive epidemiologic studies of various malformations. Another possible role of birth defects surveillance is in the identification of developmentally disabled children in need of special education, social services, and other programs.[18] The use of surveillance systems can also assist in the evaluation of programs and services, including those in which new prevention and intervention strategies, such as prenatal diagnosis and improved genetics counseling, are used.

ATTRIBUTES OF AN IDEAL BIRTH DEFECTS SURVEILLANCE SYSTEM

Population-based, Timely, and Comprehensive Case Ascertainment

The objective of collecting birth defect surveillance data is to characterize as well as possible the incidence of birth defects among the population

---

* Use of trade names is for identification only and does not constitute endorsement by the Public Health Service or the U.S. Department of Health and Human Services.

under surveillance, using available resources. The ideal birth defects system is one in which population-based information is reported in a timely manner. The timely recognition of a birth defect "epidemic" such as that resulting from the introduction of a new teratogen, depends on rapid reporting of accurate data on the occurrence of birth defects.

To minimize underreporting, case ascertainment should be comprehensive and should usually include the required review of data from multiple sources. The inclusion of personal identifiers facilitates follow-up studies and allows investigators to link infant, maternal, and paternal records. Other important characteristics for a quality birth defects surveillance system include (1) accurate and precise diagnostic criteria; (2) etiologically and pathogenetically meaningful classification schemes; (3) a large database, permitting rate comparison and analysis of trends in incidence of a relatively rare birth defect; (4) the capability to analyze the occurrence of multiple malformations; and (5) confidentiality of patient records.

Because birth defects are a heterogeneous group of conditions, accurate and precise diagnoses, as well as pathogenetically meaningful classifications, are particularly important. To better understand birth defects etiology, we need to divide birth defects into appropriate homogeneous categories.

Capacity to Analyze Multiple Malformations

The ability to analyze the occurrence of specific multiple malformations is also important. Most known teratogens are associated with a spectrum of birth defect combinations.[19-22] Many birth defects monitoring systems, however, only examine trends in rates of specific single defects, not of combinations of specific anomalies. In some instances, an increase in the rate of birth defects caused by a teratogen may be detected more rapidly by monitoring rates of defect combinations rather than by monitoring the rates of individual defects. The benefits of monitoring combinations of two and three defects have been described.[15, 23] Monitoring multiple birth defects is most effective if affected infants tend to have combinations of defects. For example, isotretinoin causes a characteristic constellation of defects, including ear malformations and central nervous system and conotruncal heart defects. The occurrence of a specific combination of these defects may be used to monitor the continued occurrence of isotretinoin embryopathy in the United States.[15]

COMPONENTS OF A BIRTH DEFECTS SURVEILLANCE SYSTEM

The components of a birth defects surveillance system include case definition and case ascertainment (including case sources and method of surveillance used to ascertain cases), as well as data collection, analysis, follow-up, and dissemination.

Case Definition

Cases to be included in the birth defects surveillance system must be clearly defined. Is any birth in which the infant has even a minor birth defect considered a case, or are cases limited to those with at least one major malformation? For example, within the Metropolitan Atlanta Congenital Defects Program (MACDP), cases include all births to residents of the five-county metropolitan Atlanta area who have at least one major birth defect detected in their first year and ascertained within their first five years of life.

Sources of Data

Multiple-source case ascertainment provides the best potential for complete case finding. Usual data sources for birth defects surveillance systems include vital records (birth and death certificates), newborn or other hospital discharge summaries, hospital records, and data from cytogenetic laboratories. Each of these sources of information has associated strengths and weaknesses.

The strengths of vital records (birth and death certificates) include (1) the complete coverage of the population (population-based), (2) the availability of some medical data, (3) the availability of some parental data, (4) the ready availability of data from previous years, (5) low cost, and (6) the potential for follow-up of birth defects cases. The weaknesses of vital records include (1) the lack of timeliness in reporting, (2) the underreporting of birth defects (information is often limited to that obtained during the newborn period), and (3) the lack of specificity of most birth defects.

The strengths of newborn hospital discharge summary data include (1) more complete recording of birth defects than with birth certificates, (2) more rapidly available data (usually within 6 months of discharge), (3) data that are already computerized and in digital form in many hospitals, and (4) the potential for follow-up of birth defects cases. Weaknesses of hospital discharge summary data include (1) a lack of maternal data, (2) a lack of access to personal identifiers (making follow-up difficult), (3) frequent difficulty in defining the population base, (4) frequent difficulty in establishing the representativeness of data, (5) incomplete recording of birth defects information, and (6) possible incomplete diagnosis in the newborn period.

The strengths of multiple source case ascertainment include (1) the relative speed of the system, (2) the relative completeness of recording, (3) more precise and accurate diagnoses, (4) relative ease for researchers to follow-up studies of cases, and (5) the availability of maternal and infant information. Weaknesses of multiple source case ascertainment include (1) high cost (often limiting the use of this method to small populations) and (2) the time needed to establish baseline data.

Passive Versus Active Surveillance

Methods of surveillance for birth defects can be subdivided into passive surveillance and active surveillance. Passive surveillance involves the identification of cases from vital records or from reports submitted to the program by staff from hospitals, clinics, or other facilities. These individuals, who may be specially trained by program staff, submit reports voluntarily or through reporting systems established by law or regulation. One example of a passive surveillance system, in which newborn hospital discharge summary data are used, is the national Birth Defects Monitoring Program (BDMP). Because BDMP investigators obtain discharge summary data from data tapes, they have no direct opportunity to review the rest of the medical record. This system is described in more detail later in this chapter.

Other examples of passive systems include systems created by legislative mandates for hospitals or physicians to report the occurrence of birth defects (as is now required in New York, New Jersey, and Nebraska), systems created by the linkage of multiple data sources (as is done in Missouri and North Carolina), and systems that are based on vital statistics data, such as the Indiana Birth Problems Registry.

Active surveillance involves the identification of cases by trained surveillance program staff who actively seek cases in hospitals, clinics, or other facilities by systematic review of medical and other records. They may also query personnel who may be knowledgeable about newly diagnosed cases. Program staff record the case information on standard forms designed for the program.

Figure 12-1 shows a summary of the status of birth defects surveillance systems within the United States. In 1991, eight states had active surveillance systems, which provided information on approximately 900,000 births (21 percent of the births in the United States that year). An additional 15 states had passive surveillance systems, which provided information on 1,445,000 births (34 percent of births) and two states had systems that were based on vital records, which provided information on 153,500 births (4 percent of births). Another four states are in implementing or planning stages.

Depending on the methods and sources of case ascertainment used, the various surveillance systems produce substantially varying birth defects rates, as shown in Table 12-1.

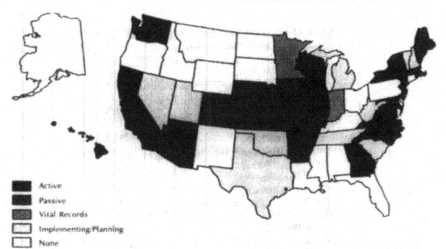

FIGURE 12-1.   Summary of the status of birth defects surveillance systems within the United States.

Data Collection

Determining what data to collect is an important aspect of birth defects surveillance. Optimally, data would include precise descriptions of all birth defects, including syndrome identification by geneticists or dysmorphologists, demographic data, pregnancy history and other birth-related data, cytogenetic and laboratory data, family history, and etiologic information. These data provide the basis for the initiation of further follow-up studies. A set of core data items, which the CDC currently recommends that workers in state birth defects surveillance programs collect, is included in the appendix to this chapter.

Data Analysis, Follow-up, and Dissemination

By monitoring birth defects surveillance data, researchers can detect differing birth defect rates in different areas as well as rate changes. The data are monitored by statistically evaluating the difference between observed and expected numbers of specific defects or defect combinations for a specified time in a specified area. Expected numbers are obtained from baseline incidence data. Such comparisons may lead to the identification of clusters of birth defects; subsequent investigation of such clusters may yield useful etiologic information.

One commonly used statistical method for monitoring birth defect trends that is now being used by MACDP is the cumulative sum (CUSUM)

TABLE 12-1   Rates of Major Birth Defects Using Various Surveillance Approaches

Method and Source	Rate[1]
Birth Certificate (NCHS[2] 1982–83)	88.9
Newborn Hospital Discharge Data (BDMP[3] 1982–85)	282.5
Mandatory Hospital Reporting Data (Nebraska 1982–85)	248.0
Linked Data Sources (Missouri 1980–84)	336.0
Active Hospital Surveillance Data (MACDP[4] 1982–87)	415.0
(Iowa 1983–86)	549.0
Physical Exam of Infant (CPP[5])	830.0

[1] per 10,000 births
[2] National Center for Health Statistics
[3] Birth Defects Monitoring Program
[4] Metropolitan Atlanta Congenital Defects Program
[5] Collaborative Perinatal Project. SOURCE: Myriantho-poulos, N.C., and C.S. Chung. Congenital Malformations. In Singletons. 1974. *Epidemiologic Survey*. Birth Defects: Orig. Art. Series, vol. X. no. 11. New York: Stratton Intercontinental Medical Book Corp.

technique. This technique involves cumulating values that are approximated by the differences between observed and expected numbers of cases.[24] When cumulative differences reach a certain specified critical level, a flag is raised for that specific defect, indicating a significant increase or decrease. These flags are based on three factors: the number of births, the defect rate expected under normal circumstances, and the average time to a flag occurring in the absence of a true underlying rate change. This last factor is commonly referred to as the average run length (ARL) to a false positive.[24] The selection of cutoff times depends on the delicate balance between sensitivity (the detection of true increases as soon as possible) and specificity (the flagging of false rate changes rarely as possible). Monitoring is often done quarterly, with researchers checking to see whether flagged defects are increasing or decreasing. Such review may lead to investigations about the nature of such changes.

Dissemination of data is another important component of a birth defects surveillance system. Routine compilation of rates and reports of changing trends or other findings is useful to health care providers and to state and local officials. Feedback is also helpful to physicians and hospital officials who assist in surveillance efforts by providing medical information.

EXAMPLES OF BIRTH DEFECTS SURVEILLANCE SYSTEMS

Metropolitan Atlanta Congenital Defects Program

The Metropolitan Atlanta Congenital Defects Program (MACDP) is a population-based birth defects surveillance system that has been in operation since 1968. MACDP is sponsored by the Georgia Mental Health Institute, Emory University School of Medicine, and the CDC. Day-to-day program operations are the responsibility of the CDC. MACDP monitors all births occurring in the five-county metropolitan Atlanta area, approximately 35,000 births each year. MACDP includes information on all live-born and stillborn infants diagnosed with at least one major birth defect within their first year of life, with diagnoses ascertained within their first five years of life.

MACDP researchers use the precise diagnosis and written description of defects collected and coded in the 6-digit MACDP code,[25] a modification of the 1977 British Paediatric Association (BPA) *Classification of Diseases*[26] and the World Health Organization's 1979 *International Classification of Diseases, 9th Revision, Clinical Modification* (IDC-9 CM).[8] Code modifications were developed by researchers from the CDC's Birth Defects and Genetic Diseases Branch. This 6-digit code permits better classification of birth defects and improves researchers' ability to study specific types of malformations.

Case ascertainment includes the review of maternal and infant medical records in multiple sources, including birth hospitals, pediatric referral hospitals, cytogenetic laboratories, and specialty clinics, as well as vital statistics from the Georgia Department of Human Resources. Multiple sources of ascertainment are used to identify potential cases. Hospital records reviewed include obstetric logs, nursery logs, pediatric logs, surgery logs, cardiac catheterization records, autopsy logs, disease indexes, and laboratory logs. The charts of all infants who are stillborn, die shortly after birth, weigh less than 2,500 grams, or are born before 37 weeks of gestational age are reviewed. Similar information from pediatric referral hospitals is reviewed, as are laboratory service records. In addition, vital statistics records (birth and death certificates) are reviewed in a search for previously unidentified cases.

MACDP case records include basic demographic information, specific written diagnoses, 6-digit codes, birth-related information, cytogenetic data, complications of birth, prenatal data, pregnancy history, family history, and other risk factor information. Birth defects rates and trends are monitored by quarterly reviews and analysis of data from MACDP. Temporal and geographic comparisons are made to search for significant changes in the rates of birth defects. Data from MACDP are published regularly by the CDC.[27]

MACDP data have been used for descriptive studies, hypothesis testing, case-control studies, family studies, and cluster investigations. Numerous epidemiologic studies have been published, including studies on Vietnam veterans' risks for fathering babies with birth defects,[10] the protective effect of periconceptional multivitamin use on the occurrence of neural tube defects,[28] maternal cocaine use as a risk factor for congenital urogenital anomalies,[29] and insulin-dependent diabetes mellitus in pregnancy and the risk of specific birth defects.[30]

Furthermore, MACDP has served as a prototype for numerous birth defects surveillance systems. MACDP researchers have encouraged the development of uniform methods of birth defects surveillance, developed a more specific coding system and a uniform set of variables for data collection, and provided a focus for collaborative studies between active surveillance systems.

Because individual birth defects are rare, researchers have difficulty in obtaining enough cases for etiologic studies. In addition, outside of the Birth Defects Monitoring Program, few national data are available on the occurrence of birth defects. The use of systems that can collaborate will substantially increase researchers' power to study relatively rare birth defects, greatly enhancing the understanding of the occurrence and etiology of birth defects. Efforts toward interstate collaboration revolve around the development of uniform methods and standards and the use of equivalent case definitions and coding systems. As an example of multisystem collaboration, the CDC's isotretinoin embryopathy surveillance efforts are focusing on state surveillance systems to provide information on the occurrence of the specific constellation of defects known to be associated with first trimester exposure to isotretinoin.[15]

Birth Defects Monitoring Program

The Birth Defects Monitoring Program (BDMP), which uses existing newborn hospital discharge databases, is the largest source of data available on newborns in the United States. Between 1982 and 1985, BDMP monitored 35 percent (1.3 million) of the total U.S. births each year for the occurrence of birth defects diagnosed during the newborn period. The monitoring program is based on two hospital information systems: the

Commission of Professional and Hospital Activities (CPHA) and the McDonnell Douglas Health Information System (MDHIS). Officials from hospitals belonging to either of these systems submit abstracted and coded discharge summary information on newborns. This information is then forwarded on computer tape to the CDC's Birth Defects and Genetic Diseases Branch for processing. Because the birth records are obtained from a nonrandom sample of U.S. hospitals, BDMP birth data are not population-based and do not constitute a random sample of all U.S. births. Data from BDMP are analyzed and reviewed quarterly to monitor the rates and trends of selected birth defects. Temporal and geographic comparisons are made to search for significant changes in rates. Data from BDMP are published regularly.[27]

In addition to allowing investigators to identify unusual trends in and rate differences between participating areas of the United States, BDMP has been useful in supporting numerous epidemiologic investigations,[31-33] including descriptive studies, follow-up studies, and program evaluations; it also has provided a starting point for case-control studies. BDMP is also an inexpensive source of national birth defects data. Because BDMP is a passive surveillance system based on hospital discharge summaries of the newborn period, the proportion of cases it detects depends on the severity of the specific defect; less severe defects can be overlooked in the newborn period, whereas more severe defects lend themselves to a prompt and accurate diagnosis. Depending on defect severity, sensitivity has been estimated to range from 10 to 98 percent.[27] Although sensitivity may be low for certain defects, BDMP has proven useful while remaining simple, flexible, and well-accepted. The number of participating hospitals, however, continues to decline each year. CDC researchers are investigating new avenues for national birth defects surveillance, including collaboration among state birth defects monitoring programs.

INTERNATIONAL ACTIVITIES

International Clearinghouse for Birth Defects Monitoring Systems

The International Clearinghouse for Birth Defects Monitoring Systems (ICBDMS) was founded in 1974 as a means of communicating birth defects data from surveillance systems from around the world.[34] ICBDMS is an independent, nonprofit organization that is affiliated with the World Health Organization. Information is shared among 26 member programs, including MACDP, BDMP, and systems in the European community and elsewhere. Information on birth defects is available on more than 4.5 million births each year from 30 countries. Some of the participating programs are nationwide, population-based, and mandated by legislation, whereas others are hospital-based research programs. Because of the differences among these programs, completeness of ascertainment, diagnostic criteria, and other factors contribute to the extent to which birth defects are reported. The primary purpose of the ICBDMS, however, is to detect changes in birth defects rates. For this purpose, completeness of ascertainment is of secondary importance, provided ascertainment procedures remain stable over time. ICBDMS participants exchange data through quarterly reports and prepare an annual report for publication.[34] ICBDMS covers only a fraction of the world's births, and the sample is unrepresentative of the world's population as a whole. ICBDMS participants encourage the formation and participation of other monitoring programs in the hope of more representative coverage of the world's population.

On the initiative of ICBDMS and at the invitation of the Norwegian government, the International Centre for Birth Defects (ICBD) has recently been established at the University of Bergen, Norway.[35] The purpose of ICBD is to promote and advance ICBDM's main objective, which is the prevention of birth defects. ICBD engages in scientific research, conducts surveillance, and prepares statistics by working closely with ICBDM member programs.[35] One goal of ICBD is to broaden international contacts with organizations concerned with the study and prevention of birth defects.

Eurocat

The European Registers of Congenital Abnormalities and Twins (EUROCAT) program is a concerted action project of the European Economic Community.[36] Program participants began recording data in 1979. Surveillance of birth defects is accomplished through a network of 20 coordinated regional registries. The goal of each registry is to report all cases of birth defects, chromosomal abnormalities, and metabolic disorders occurring among babies born to women living in well-defined geographic regions. Epidemiologic data are recorded on live births, stillbirths, and induced terminations. In each of the participating centers, multisource case ascertainment is used, including birth and death certificates, maternity and hospital records, cytogenetic reports, pathology services data, and maternal and child health services data.[37] Participating registries use the British Paediatric Association *Classification of Diseases.*[26]

SPECIAL CONSIDERATIONS FOR DEVELOPING COUNTRIES

In developing countries, birth defects are usually not the leading cause of infant mortality,[38] although rates of some birth defects are actually higher than in developed countries.[39] With their wide variation in ethnic, cultural, political, and economic situations, developing countries would benefit from the expansion of current birth defects surveillance activities. Developing countries could potentially be more exposed to new teratogens because of relative failures in their systems to regulate such exposures.[38] Likewise, many developing populations are more likely to be immunologically unprotected from rubella, suffer from malnutrition, have advanced reproductive ages, and be exposed to environmental, agricultural, and industrial pollutants.[38]

In the face of limited resources, surveillance systems in developing countries should be implemented by using existing organizations to the fullest extent possible. Useful systems can be started as a limited activity within a few large maternity hospitals or within a single city and expanded later as resources permit. Officials have recommended that such systems in developing countries begin as hospital-based systems, relying on information voluntarily reported by a limited number of health care providers.[38] These systems may overcome some of the usual limitations found in developing countries, including political and institutional instability, and the lack of reliable vital and health statistics.

CONCLUDING REMARKS

In the United States, birth defects are the leading cause of infant mortality and the fifth leading cause of years of potential life lost. Because of the relative rarity of individual defects, surveillance systems must continue to expand. To maximize the capability of these systems to interact, researchers need to collect, ascertain, and code data using consistent methods. In addition, health officials in areas lacking in birth defects surveillance activities should be encouraged to use the available resources to the greatest extent possible.

The Year 2000 Objectives[40] outline the necessity for the implementation and coordination of birth defects surveillance. Such programs can play an important role in defining problems and evaluating prevention programs. Adverse reproductive outcomes in general can be reduced through combined efforts at the international, federal, state, and local levels through the use of voluntary organizations, business and industry, and the health professions.

The development of a uniform approach to the collection and analysis of data through various surveillance programs is a major challenge. Responding to that challenge will help contribute to our knowledge of the causes of birth defects, develop strategies to prevent them, and assist in the evaluation and delivery of services to children born with birth defects.

Notes
1. Centers for Disease Control. 1989. Contribution of birth defects to infant mortality: United States, 1986. *MMWR* 38:633–635.
2. Centers for Disease Control. 1990. Years of potential life lost before ages 65 and 85: United States, 1987 and 1988. *MMWR* 39:20–22.
3. Edmonds, L. D., P. M. Layde, L. M. James, J. W. Flynt, J. D. Erickson, and G. P. Oakley, Jr. 1981. Congenital malformations surveillance: two American systems. *Int J Epidemiol* 10(3):247–252.
4. Lynberg, M. C., M. J. Khoury, and G. P. Oakley, Jr. 1989. The contribution of birth defects to infant mortality: United States, 1986. Paper presented at the American Public Health Association 117th Annual Meeting, October 22–26, Chicago, Illinois.
5. Hall, J. G., E. K. Powers, R. T. McIlvaine, and V. H. Ean. 1978. The frequency and financial burden of genetic disease in a pediatric hospital. *Am J Med Genet* 1:417–436.
6. Epstein, C. J. Genetic disorders and birth defects. In: Rudolph A. M., J. I. E. Hoffman, and S. Axelrod, eds. 1987. *Pediatrics,* 209–210. Norwalk, Conn.: Appleton & Lange.
7. Centers for Disease Control. 1989. Economic burden of spina bifida: United States, 1980–1990. *MMWR* 38:264–267.
8. World Health Organization. 1979. *International Classification of Diseases, 9th Revision.* Geneva: World Health Organization.
9. Spranger, J., K. Benirschke, J. G. Hall et al. 1982. Errors of morphogenesis: concepts and terms recommendations of an international working group. *J Pediatr* 100:160–165.
10. Erickson, J. D., J. Mulinare, P. W. McClain et al. 1984. Vietnam veterans' risk for fathering babies with birth defects. *JAMA* 252:903–912.
11. Kallen, B., S. Hay, and M. Klingberg. Birth defects monitoring systems accomplishments and goals. In: Kalter, H., ed. 1984. *Issues and Reviews in Teratology,* 2:1–22. New York/London: Plenum Publishing Corp.
12. Holtzman, N. A., and M. J. Khoury. 1986. Monitoring for congenital malformations. *Ann Rev Public Health* 7:237–266.
13. May, P. A., and K. J. Hymbaugh. 1989. A macro-level fetal alcohol syndrome prevention program for Native Americans and Alaska natives: description and evaluation. *J Stud Alcohol* 50:508–518.
14. Kaplan, K. M., S. L. Cochi, L. D. Edmonds et al. 1990. A profile of mothers giving birth to infants with congenital rubella syndrome: an assessment of risk factors. *Am J Dis Child* 144:118–123.
15. Lynberg, M. C., M. J. Khoury, E. J. Lammer et al. 1990. Sensitivity, specificity, and positive predictive value of multiple malformations in isotretinoin embryopathy surveillance. *Teratology* 42:513–519.
16. Mili, F., M. J. Khoury, W. D. Flanders, and R. S. Greenberg. 1990. Risk of childhood cancer for infants with birth defects: a record-linkage study, 1968–1988 (abstract). *Am J Epidemiol* 132:764–765.
17. Baird, P. A., and A. D. Sadovnick. 1988. Life expectancy in Down's syndrome adults. *Lancet* 2:1354–1356.

18. Miller, J. R. 1977. Birth defects monitoring systems: overview. *Congenital Anomalies* 17:1–12.

19. Sever, J. L. and R. L. Brent, eds. 1986. *Teratogen Update: Environmentally Induced Birth Defects Risks.* New York: Alan R. Liss.

20. Shepard, T. H. 1986. *Catalog of Teratogenic Agents.* 5th ed. Baltimore: Johns Hopkins University Press.

21. Schardein, J. L. 1985. *Chemically Induced Birth Defects.* New York: Marcel Dekker.

22. Jones, K. L. 1988. *Smith's Recognizable Patterns of Human Malformation.* 4th ed. Philadelphia: W.B. Saunders Company.

23. Khoury, M. J., M. M. Adams, P. Rhodes, and J. D. Erickson. 1987. Monitoring for multiple malformations in the detection of epidemics of birth defects. *Teratology* 36:345–354.

24. Lucas, J. M. 1985. Counted data cusums. *Technometrics* 27:129–144.

25. Centers for Disease Control. 1989. *Metropolitan Atlanta Congenital Defects Program Procedure Manual.* Atlanta, Ga.: CDC.

26. British Paediatric Association. 1977. *Classification of Diseases.* London: The British Paediatric Association.

27. Centers for Disease Control. In press. *Congenital Malformations Surveillance Report.* Atlanta, Ga.: CDC.

28. Mulinare, J., J. F. Cordero, J. D. Erickson, and R. J. Berry. 1988. Periconceptional use of multivitamins and the occurrence of neural tube defects. *JAMA* 260:3141–3145.

29. Chavez, G. F., J. Mulinare, and J. F. Cordero. 1989. Maternal cocaine use during early pregnancy as a risk factor for congenital urogenital anomalies. *JAMA* 262(6):795–798.

30. Becerra, J. E., M. J. Khoury, J. F. Cordero, and J. D. Erickson. 1988. Insulin-dependent diabetes mellitus in pregnancy and the risk for specific birth defects. *Pediatr Res* 23:266A.

31. Stroup, N. E., L. D. Edmonds, and T. R. O'Brien. 1990. Renal agenesis and dysgenesis: are they increasing? *Teratology* 42:383–395.

32. Edmonds, L. D., C. E. Anderson, J. W. Flynt, Jr., and L. M. James. 1978. Congenital central nervous system malformations and vinyl chloride monomer exposure: a community study. *Teratology* 17:137–142.

33. Cochi, S. L., L. E. Edmonds, K. Dyer et al. 1989. Congenital rubella syndrome in the United States, 1970–1985: on the verge of elimination. *Am J Epidemiol* 129:349–361.

34. International Clearinghouse for Birth Defects Monitoring Systems: Annual Report, 1987. ISSN 0743-5703.

35. Anonymous. 1990. Announcements. *Teratology* 42:102.

36. Lechat, M. F., ed. 1989. *Eurocat Report: Surveillance of Congenital Anomalies, Years 1980–1986.* Brussels: Department of Epidemiology, Catholic University of Louvain.

37. Lechat, M. F., ed. 1986. *Eurocat Report: Surveillance of Congenital Anomalies, Years 1980–1983.* Brussels: Department of Epidemiology, Catholic University of Louvain.

38. Castillo, E. E. Unpublished. Guidelines for the formation of national programmes for the prevention and control of congenital anomalies in developing countries.
39. Kallen, B., and L. Knudsen. 1989. Effect of maternal age distribution and prenatal diagnosis on the population rates of Down's syndrome: a comparative study of nineteen populations. *Hereditas* 110:55–60.
40. Healthy People 2000: National Health Promotion and Disease Prevention Objectives DHHS PHS, September 1990. U.S. Dept. of Health and Human Services Publication No. (PHS) 91-50213 U.S. Government Printing Office, Washington, D.C.

APPENDIX

A Recommended Set of Core Data Items for Collection by State Birth Defects Surveillance Programs

Presented at the 116th Annual Meeting of the American Public Health Association, Boston, Massachusetts November 13–17, 1988

Larry D. Edmonds, Helen B. Mackley, Mark C. Fulcomer, Susan R. Panny, and F. John Meaney

Data Item	Recommended Level of Inclusion	Recommended Use of Data	Recommended by NCHS*
I. Infant			
A. Date of birth (month, day, year)	Recommended	National	Yes
B. Sex (male, female, ambiguous, unknown)	Recommended	National	Yes
C. Race (generated from parents)	Optional	National	Yes
D. Ethnicity (collected separately from race)	Optional	National	Yes
E. Name (including any alias)	Recommended	State	Yes
F. Unique health I.D.	Optional	State	No
G. Date of report (month, day, year)	Recommended	National	Yes
H. Source of report (name, phone)	Recommended	National	Yes
I. Residence			
1. Mother at infant's birth			
City/county/state	Recommended	National	Yes
Zip code	Recommended	National	Yes
Census tract (derived from address)	Optional	State	No
2. Mother at conception	Optional	National	No
J. Place of birth			
1. Country	Recommended	National	Yes
2. City	Recommended	National	Yes
3. State	Recommended	National	Yes
4. County	Recommended	National	Yes
5. Zip code	Recommended	National	No
6. Name of hospital/code	Recommended	State	Yes

K. Pregnancy outcome		
1. Liveborn	Recommended	National	Yes
2. Stillborn >20 weeks	Recommended	National	Yes
3. Induced abortion	Optional	National	Yes
4. Spontaneous abortion	Optional	National	Yes
5. Unknown abortion	Optional	National	Yes
L. Birthweight in grams	Recommended	National	Yes
M. Apgar	Optional	National	Yes
N. Plurality	Recommended	National	Yes
O. Gestational age			
1. By last menstrual period	Recommended	National	Yes
2. By newborn examination	Optional	National	Yes
3. By ultrasound	Optional	National	No
P. Diagnosis (descriptions of all defects)	Recommended	National	No
Q. Source and place of diagnosis	Optional	National	No
R. Date of each diagnosis	Recommended	National	No
S. Date of death (month, day, year)	Recommended	National	Yes
T. Place of death			
1. Country	Recommended	National	Yes
2. City/state/county	Recommended	National	Yes
3. Zip code	Recommended	National	Yes
4. Name of hospital/code	Optional	State	Yes
U. Cytogenetic studies			
1. Performed (yes, no, unknown)	Recommended	National	No
2. Results	Optional	National	No

*National Center for Health Statistics

(Continued on next page)

Data Item	Recommended Level of Inclusion	Recommended Use of Data	Recommended by NCHS*
V. Autopsy			
1. Performed (yes, no, unknown)	Recommended	National	Yes
2. Results	Optional	National	No
W. Physicians of record			
1. Pediatrician/obstetrician/family physician (name, phone)	Recommended	State	No
II. Mother			
A. Date of birth (month, day, year)	Recommended	National	Yes
B. Race	Recommended	National	Yes
C. Ethnicity (collected separately from race)	Optional	National	Yes
D. Name (including maiden surname for matching)	Recommended	State	Yes
E. Unique health I.D.	Optional	State	No
F. Occupation			
1. Usual	Optional	National	No
2. At time of conception or during first trimester	Optional	National	No
G. Education	Recommended	National	Yes
H. Method of payment	Optional	National	No
I. Summary totals of mother's previous pregnancies			
1. Total of previous pregnancies	Recommended	National	Yes
2. Live births	Recommended	National	Yes
3. Stillbirths >20 weeks	Recommended	National	No
4. Spontaneous abortions	Recommended	National	No
5. Induced abortions	Recommended	National	No

	Recommended / Optional	National / State	Yes / No
6. Neonatal deaths	Recommended	National	No
7. Post-neonatal deaths	Recommended	National	No
8. Total of pregnancies with malformations	Optional	National	No
J. Risk factors for the current pregnancy			
1. Complications during pregnancy	Recommended	National	Yes
2. Illness or conditions during pregnancy	Recommended	National	Yes
3. Complications of labor and delivery	Optional	National	Yes
4. Method of delivery	Optional	National	Yes
5. Month prenatal care began	Optional	National	Yes
6. Number of prenatal visits	Optional	National	Yes
7. Parentally-identified teratogenic exposures	Optional	National	No
8. Use of tobacco	Optional	National	Yes
9. Use of alcohol	Optional	National	Yes
10. Use of nonprescription drugs	Optional	National	No
11. Prenatal diagnostic procedures	Optional	National	Yes
12. Family history of malformations	Optional	National	No
III. Father			
A. Date of birth (month, day, year)	Recommended	National	Yes
B. Race	Recommended	National	Yes
C. Ethnicity (collected separately from race)	Optional	National	Yes
D. Name	Optional	State	Yes
E. Unique health I.D.	Optional	State	No
F. Occupation			
1. Usual	Optional	National	No
2. At time of conception or during first trimester	Optional	National	No
G. Education	Optional	National	Yes

* National Center for Health Statistics

13

Surveillance of Occupational Illness and Injury

Edward L. Baker and Thomas P. Matte

GENERAL PRINCIPLES

To be effective, surveillance must be directly linked to preventive action. In the case of occupational health, the actions prompted by the surveillance system should be directed not only at the individual case or the affected group, but also at the responsible workplace factors. Surveillance programs (i.e., secondary prevention) should be designed to support programs to control workplace hazards (i.e., primary prevention). In occupational safety and health, a surveillance program should (1) identify cases of occupational illness or injury, and/or (2) monitor trends of occupational illness or injury.

The purpose of case identification is to target an intervention of direct value to the affected individual and to others at risk of developing the same disorder. Case identification is followed by attempts to identify other individuals at risk and to control environmental factors that are responsible for disease etiology. Case identification occurs in three types of surveillance programs: (1) medical screening, (2) health care provider reporting, and (3) employer case reporting.

Surveillance programs in the workplace can also be used to monitor trends of illness, injury, or exposure to workplace hazards. In such activity, surveillance data are developed to assess variations in rates between (1) different industrial groups, (2) different geographic areas, and/or (3) different time periods. From such comparisons, health officials can identify target industries or geographic areas requiring further investigation or intervention. In this way, surveillance of health or exposure trends is used to evaluate the efficacy of programs designed to control occupational hazards.

Surveillance of occupational disease and injury can involve the monitoring of either health effects among the general workforce, or hazards present in the workplace. In many situations, surveillance of individual health effects or workplace hazards alone may be useful. Linkage of the data derived from health effects and hazard surveillance for the same population is even more desirable.

In surveillance of health effects, a system may target the actual health event (i.e., the occurrence of an occupational injury or the diagnosis of a case of an occupational illness) or a change in a biological function of an exposed individual (e.g., loss of pulmonary function or disruption of heme metabolism). For surveillance purposes, occupational illnesses can be divided into two groups: (1) disorders caused primarily by a single occupational exposure or hazard, (such as lead poisoning or silicosis); and (2) disorders of multifactorial etiology for which occupational factors may serve as one of several causal factors (such as lung cancer). Further, occupational hazards may exacerbate a preexisting health condition.

Surveillance of disorders caused by a single exposure or hazard can be accomplished by specifying the condition and developing an approach to evaluating the health status of the worker and the worker's exposure history. Such diseases, caused primarily by a single occupational exposure or hazard, are termed "occupational diseases" by the World Health Organization (WHO).

Surveillance of multifactorial diseases for which occupational factors may play a contributing role is often not useful. Surveillance is made difficult by problems in diagnosis of the condition or in ascertainment of the relative importance of nonoccupational factors in disease etiology. Control of such conditions is best accomplished by relying upon primary control of the offending hazard through environmental measures, and through the performance of hazard surveillance to monitor the effectiveness of such controls.

Hazard surveillance consists of periodic characterization of chemical or physical hazards in the workplace. Such characterization can be accomplished by the direct measurement of airborne contaminants using industrial hygiene procedures or by indirect approaches to an assessment of the degree of hazard present in the work environment. Since many chemical, physical, and biological agents have been found to present a significant hazard to the health of workers, surveillance of the occurrences of hazards provides very useful information even in the absence of simultaneous health status assessment. In many industries, certain types of hazard surveillance (i.e., direct measurement of levels of airborne contaminants or noise level) are used to direct strategies for primary prevention.

CONDUCT OF SURVEILLANCE

Medical Screening

Medical screening is the administration of a medical test for the purpose of detecting organ dysfunction or disease before the person would normally seek medical care and at a time when intervention is beneficial. Screening tests may indicate the presence of a disease, or merely a higher probability of disease and the need for additional, confirmatory testing.

If performed correctly, conduct of an occupational health screening program is one of the most complex processes in medical practice.[1] In designing the program, the practitioner must be familiar with clinical medicine and toxicology, and understand the importance of a standardized approach to data collection. In analyzing and interpreting the data, the practitioner must be familiar with epidemiology and clinical decision analysis, and understand the applicability of industrial hygiene exposure measurements. In making recommendations based on these interpretations, the practitioner must take cognizance of existing laws and regulations and act ethically in situations in which conflicts of interest often exist. Finally, screening tests have certain operational characteristics (i.e., sensitivity, specificity, predictive value, and reliability) that should be considered in designing and evaluating workplace medical programs.

Surveillance versus Screening: A Few Words on Terminology

As described in this text, the term "surveillance" encompasses a broad range of activities which include monitoring the results of screening. The term "medical surveillance" in standards promulgated by the Occupational Safety and Health Administration (OSHA) corresponds reasonably well in usage to the term "screening." The process of "medical surveillance" or "screening" involves direct medical evaluations of individuals at risk for the development of certain disorders.

Purposes of Medical Screening

The main focus of workplace medical examination programs should be screening to benefit individual workers.[2] In the workplace context, screening tests are used to identify toxic health effects at an earlier stage than they would be identified without screening. Target conditions should be those for which interventions—reducing worker exposure to the offending agent and/or medical treatment—are more beneficial when applied early

TABLE 13-1   **Process of Designing and Implementing a Screening Program**

---

1. Assessment of Workplace Hazards
2. Identification of Target Organ Toxicities for Each Hazard
3. Selection of Test for Each "Screenable Health Effect"
4. Development of Action Criteria
5. Standardization of Data Collection Process
6. Performance of Testing
7. Interpretation of Test Results
8. Test Confirmation
9. Determination of Work Status
10. Notification
11. Diagnostic Evaluation
12. Evaluation and Control of Exposure
13. Recordkeeping

---

in the disease process. Thus, the principal objective of workplace medical screening is secondary prevention of disease in the people who are screened. Screening can also be used to establish the work-relatedness of a previously diagnosed condition and to generate data for use in the surveillance of groups of workers.

Biological monitoring is the measurement and assessment of workplace agents or their metabolites in biological specimens (for example, blood, urine, or hair) to evaluate exposure and absorption by all routes (i.e., inhalation, percutaneous, or ingestion). Biological monitoring results, collected as part of a screening program, can be used to supplement the results of exposure monitoring.

A General Approach to the Performance of Screening Programs

The design and conduct of a screening program should follow 13 steps (see Table 13-1).[3] In addition to following these steps to screen individuals, the data collected can be aggregated for an analysis of the health status of a group with similar risks.

Step 1: Hazard Assessment

Exposure levels and routes of absorption of the substances in the work environment should be ascertained to assess individual worker risk. Situations where exposure mixtures are seen and in which workload varies widely complicate the process of hazard assessment considerably.

Step 2: Identification of Target Organ Toxicity

From occupational medicine texts such as this book, potential toxicity for each significant workplace hazard can be identified. Often such information is limited, particularly with respect to meaningful human dose-response data. Recommendations of NIOSH or regulations promulgated by OSHA are often based on data which are limited in this regard.

Step 3: Selection of Tests

For a health effect to be "screenable," a test must be available that can detect the toxic health effect before it would normally cause a worker to present for medical attention (i.e., during the "preclinical" phase), and at a time when intervention (reduction of exposure and/or medical treatment) is more beneficial than for more advanced disease. Generally, the preclinical phase of an effect must be of sufficient duration (at least weeks or months) to be detected by a screening test given at feasible intervals. Screening is of little help in preventing acute, severe health effects, such as cyanide poisoning, since the preclinical phase is too brief to be detected. Some acute, but intermittent health effects, such as solvent intoxication, may be amenable to screening by questionnaire, since workers may recall symptomatic episodes at screening examinations weeks or months after they occur. This information may be useful, since such episodes may precede the development of chronic central nervous system toxicity.

Test selection should also be governed by the considerations of sensitivity, specificity, predictive value, and reliability as defined above. Often tests used in clinical practice are found to be inadequate if considered in this way.

Step 4: Development of Action Criteria

When the medical evaluation of workers is undertaken, the health professional designing the program should have a plan for how medical data will be interpreted and acted upon. This plan should include criteria to determine when action will be taken in response to medical test results. To assist in the interpretation of results of some screening tests, guidelines have been developed by consensus groups. These guidelines exist primarily for biological monitoring tests, such as the biological exposure index (BEI) developed by the American Conference of Governmental Industrial Hygienists (ACGIH). In certain OSHA Standards, guidelines are provided for the interpretation of such tests (e.g., blood lead levels). Guidance in the interpretation of the significance of other tests can also be found in selected OSHA Standards (e.g., pulmonary function testing in the Cotton Dust Standard). Unfortunately, guidance is limited and inconsistent. For this and other reasons, OSHA has proposed a generic approach to medical surveillance which would create a more comprehensive and uniform approach to this complex process.

Pending the development of more comprehensive guidance, practitioners should establish, for their programs, criteria for action that apply to each test. In developing these criteria, practitioners should evaluate testing data to determine action levels that are statistically appropriate and biologically meaningful.

Step 5: Standardization of Testing Process
Staff should be trained in the proper performance of tests so that the results will be intelligible. If adequate systems of quality control do not exist, data integrity over time cannot be assured. Therefore, use of quality control systems and standardized tests is essential for optimum reliability and comparability.

Step 6: Test Performance
Testing should be performed on a voluntary basis. Employees should be provided with information regarding the risks and benefits of testing and with written evidence of informed consent to testing. Confidentiality of records should be protected through the development of a record access control system that ensures that only those who need to know the results will have access to them.

Step 7: Interpretation of Test Results
Test interpretation should be based on pre-determined action criteria, exposure data provided by the employer, and the presence of potentially unfounding nonoccupational factors. Test interpretation is the responsibility of the medical practitioner, not the employer.

Step 8: Test Confirmation
Abnormal test results should be confirmed immediately before further action is taken. At the discretion of the person responsible for directing the program, the employee may be removed from exposure pending results of confirmatory testing.

Step 9: Determination of Work Fitness
The proper use of medical testing in determining whether a worker should be removed from a hazardous job has received considerable attention and is subject to a proportional amount of controversy. If continued work exposure may further compromise the health of the worker, the worker should be removed from exposure pending the resolution of the health problem or the abatement of the offending hazard. Since retention of salary

and benefits often does not occur following such "medical removal," OSHA has required under certain conditions—for instance, lead exposure—that employers not reduce or terminate wages and benefits following such a transfer. Under a generic OSHA standard or medical screening, such wage and benefit protection could be extended to all situations where job transfer occurs due to a medical determination.

Step 10: Notification
Frequently, employees do not receive notification of the results of medical screening tests. Such notification should be prompt and informative, and strict confidentiality procedures should be followed. The implications of the test results should be explained by a qualified health professional in a manner that is clearly understood by the employee.

Step 11: Diagnostic Evaluation
Screening tests rarely, if ever, provide a definitive diagnosis, and abnormal results should be evaluated according to good medical practice. In some instances, further investigation may be limited to a more detailed medical history to clarify symptoms reported on a questionnaire. In other cases, referral to a specialist may be required. The action plan should include conditions under which such referrals are indicated.

Step 12: Evaluation and Control of Exposure
When a toxic effect is established or strongly suspected from medical test results, the most important action is to initiate a reevaluation of the work environment of the affected employee and, if indicated, to implement modifications to reduce exposure to levels that are safe for the affected person. In such instances, notification of the employer is necessary. However, employers should only be provided with information that is relevant and necessary for evaluation and modification of the work environment, and every effort should be made to keep medical data confidential, to the extent feasible.

Once an employer has been notified of a screening result requiring an evaluation of the environment, a sequence of measures should be followed until the problem is resolved. These should include the measurement of airborne levels, the assessment of control measures such as ventilation systems and personal protective equipment, modifications in control measures as appropriate, and the assessment of the effectiveness of the modifications.

Once environmental modifications have been effected, it is again necessary to determine whether the worker can safely return to or remain in the exposed job. When an affected person is returned to an exposed job, frequent, ongoing medical evaluation may be recommended. Whenever an examining physician recommends that an employee be removed from an exposed job, the employee should be informed of the basis for the recommendation; namely, the risk and severity of an adverse outcome if the employee remains in the exposed job.

Step 13: Recordkeeping

Medical records should include examination results, interpretations, and documentation of employee and employer notifications. In addition, employers should keep records of notifications they have received of adverse effects detected by screening, and of exposure evaluations/modifications carried out in response to such notifications.

INTERPRETATION AND ACTION BASED ON GROUP TEST RESULTS

Results from individuals with similar exposure situations can be pooled to evaluate group health status. Such an evaluation is useful in assessing the efficacy of control measures. At times, group analyses may reveal important information that is not provided by individual analyses alone. The procedure for performing such analyses is described in standard epidemiology and biostatistical texts. The process of applying epidemiological principles to occupational health screening data is also described in other books. Practitioners have a responsibility to perform group analyses of screening data, since such analyses can identify potential breakdowns in hazard control programs before they would be evident from individual data.

Legal and Ethical Responsibilities

Physician Responsibilities

Screening programs should be designed by and administered under the direction of a licensed physician, preferably one with training in occupational medicine. The physician has a responsibility both to the employee being screened and to the employer.[4] If these responsibilities generate conflicting courses of action, the physician's responsibility to the employee takes precedence in determining the course of action. The American College of Occupational Medicine's Code of Ethics provides direct guidance in such difficult situations.

Physicians should provide all medical test results to the employee, along with an interpretation of the "abnormal" tests.[5] The physician also has a responsibility to see that appropriate medical follow-up of abnormal test results occur. Further, the physician has a responsibility to the employee to see that, if worksite exposures were responsible for abnormal test findings, these exposures are controlled to an acceptable level before the employee returns to work.

Finally, the physician should ascertain whether the employee's coworkers with similar exposures are at risk and, if so, appropriate action should be taken (e.g., screening). When a physician recommends that an employee be removed from a particular job because of health risks from further exposure, he or she should inform the employee of the basis of his or her recommendation, including any uncertainty about the benefits of removal.

Physicians should provide to the management of the company only the information that is needed to guide management actions. In situations where the medical department is part of the company (i.e., "in-house"), specific procedures should be developed in order to control access to medical information by personnel offices and by other company personnel. Medical results should be released to management if such knowledge would prompt action by management to control a hazardous exposure or to act in other specific ways to protect the health of employees. In such situations, the employee should be informed that disclosure will take place.

Employer Responsibilities

In addition to providing unrestricted access to medical screening for employees at risk, employers should provide information to the responsible physician and should act on the results of tests when a workplace factor is implicated. Exposure information (for example, job history, results of environmental sampling) should be provided to the physician. Information about applicable OSHA Standards, material safety data sheets, and the extent of the use of personal protective equipment should also be provided. Finally, the employer has the primary responsibility for maintaining a safe and healthful workplace.

Employee Responsibilities

As in any medical evaluation, employees are responsible for providing accurate information (e.g., medical history) and for cooperating with medical testing procedures (e.g., providing full effort on pulmonary function testing). In those instances where individual behavior—including either job practices or personal habits—contributes to the development of a health problem, the individual should assume personal responsibility for changing the behavior to reduce the risk.

TABLE 13-2   **Substances Requiring Medical Surveillance by OSHA Standards**

2-acetylaminofluorene	ethylene oxide
acrylonitrile	ethyleneimine
4-aminodiphenyl	formaldehyde
inorganic arsenic	hazardous waste
asbestos	lead
benzene	methyl chloromethyl
benzidine	ether
bis-chloromethyl ether	alpha-naphthylamine
coal tar pitch volatiles	beta-naphthylamine
coke oven emissions	4-nitrobiphenyl
cotton dust	n-nitrosodimethylamine
dibromochloropropane	noise
3,3'-dichlorobenzidine	beta-propiolactone
4-dimethylaminoazobenzene	

OSHA Requirements

Under existing OSHA Standards, employers are required to provide employees with access to medical screening examination under a variety of circumstances (see Table 13-2). In a few instances, decision models are provided (e.g., lead and cotton dust standards) to help guide physicians in their evaluation of results and in their recommendations for action. In most instances, little or no guidance is provided in the interpretation of results. OSHA requires that records be maintained for the duration of employment plus 30 years and that access of the employee to his or her personal records should be granted upon request.

HEALTH CARE PROVIDER
CASE REPORTING

Across the nation, regulations have been issued by state departments of health or departments of labor that instruct health care providers to report suspect cases of occupational illness or injury to an office of state government.[6] In some states, consultation services are made available to the employer to assist in the investigation and remediation of the suspect causes of a case report. Requirements for reporting vary widely from state to state, and are not well publicized within the medical community. Further, health care providers often fail to report since, at times, no action is taken in follow-up to the report.

To develop a systematic approach to the utilization of reports from health care providers, the National Institute for Occupational Safety and

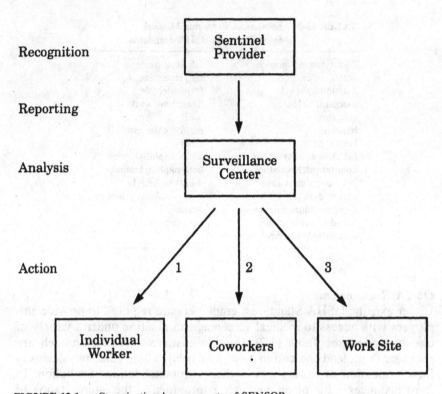

Recognition

Reporting

Analysis

Action

FIGURE 13-1.   Organizational components of SENSOR.

Health (NIOSH) recently developed the Sentinel Event Notification System for Occupational Risks (SENSOR)[7] (see Fig. 13-1). The system, now operating in approximately ten states, consists of a network of sentinel health care providers linked to the state health department. In addition to developing a network of providers, the health department determines which conditions should be reported. Most of the conditions targeted by states are drawn from a list developed by NIOSH:

1. Carpal tunnel syndrome
2. Lead poisoning
3. Noise-induced hearing loss
4. Occupational asthma
5. Pesticide poisoning
6. Silicosis

For each condition, reporting guidelines were developed to facilitate recognition of the case by the provider. Once reports are received and confirmed by the health department's surveillance centers, an active response occurs. Three possible actions may take place: (1) management of the individual case, (2) screening of coworkers with similar job exposure, and/or (3) investigation of the worksite.

Employer Case Reporting

As previously mentioned, employers are required by OSHA to record occurrences of occupational illness and injury on a form maintained at the worksite ("the OSHA log"). The responsibility for completing this record often falls to an individual without medical training and guidance in determining what should be recorded. Studies have shown that many disorders, particularly occupational illnesses, are not reported in the OSHA log.[8]

Each year, the Bureau of Labor Statistics of the U.S. Department of Labor collects a sample of these records from a portion of U.S. employers; certain categories of the workforce are not included in the survey. This sample is used to generate national estimates for selected conditions.

MONITORING INJURY, ILLNESS, AND EXPOSURE TRENDS

General Considerations

Surveillance systems designed to monitor trends for occupational disorders or exposure usually rely on existing records collected for purposes other than surveillance.[9] These records are then coded or modified in some way to make them suitable for analysis. Each data source has certain limitations and advantages that must be considered in assessing the usefulness of the data sources for surveillance purposes.

Pre-existing Health Care and Vital Records

Many types of health records contain diagnostic information on conditions appropriate for surveillance. Death certificates (including those on fetal deaths), birth certificates, hospital discharge records, office records of health care providers, and insurance claim files represent potential data sources for surveillance activities. Limitations include (1) information on the occupation of the patient is often not in the record, and (2) physicians often fail to recognize disorders caused by occupational hazards. Advantages include (1) records are available at modest cost, and (2) records are coded using generally accepted code schemes (e.g., International Classification of Disease). The process of using health care provider records in

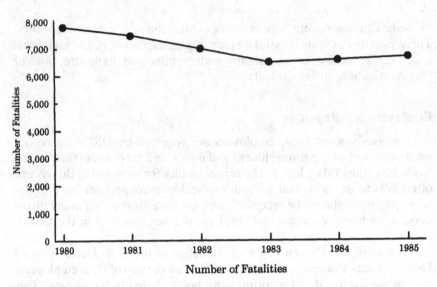

FIGURE 13-2.   Traumatic occupational fatality totals by year, 1980–1985.

surveillance may serve to improve awareness among health care providers of the impact of work on health.

In summary, health care records, if collected and coded, can be useful sources of surveillance data, particularly in the case of death certificates which contain information on the occupation of the deceased person. An excellent example of the utility of death certificates in monitoring trends of fatal occupational injury is the NIOSH National Traumatic Occupational Fatality (NTOF) database.[10] Currently, this database contains the records of all U.S. occupational fatalities from 1980 to 1985; data from subsequent years are being added. The NTOF data show a decline in the rate of occupational fatalities over the 6-year period (Figure 13-2) and an alarmingly high proportion of homicides occurring at work among females. Finally, the data show that the highest fatality rates occur in four industries: mining, transportation, construction, and agriculture (Figure 13-3).

Workers' Compensation Data

Each state in the U.S. maintains a workers' compensation system that generates data of potential use in surveillance. To be entered into the system, a worker must recognize his or her condition as work-related and file a claim. To receive compensation, the worker must also satisfy state regulations for eligibility, and successfully win a decision by the workers' compensation board.

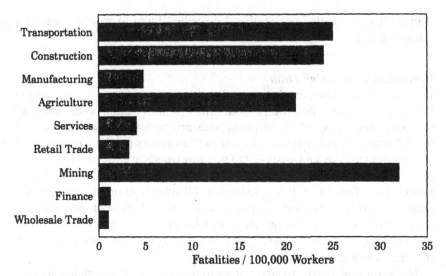

FIGURE 13-3.   Traumatic occupational fatality rates by industrial division, 1980–1985.

Limitations of workers' compensation data for surveillance are: 1) workers' compensation data will consistently underestimate the true rate of occurrence of occupational disorders. Furthermore, the rate of underestimation will vary between and among conditions, with greater underreporting for diseases than for occupational injuries. 2) Many workers' compensation systems require that claims be filed within a brief time period (e.g., one year) following the suspect exposure; this requirement essentially prevents filing claims for occupational diseases of long latency such as cancer.

Nevertheless, there are significant advantages to using workers' compensation data, including (1) all records in the data set relate to conditions of suspected occupational etiology; (2) information on the job and industry for each claimant is contained in the record; (3) the circumstances of the illness or injury are frequently described in a way that provides understanding of the cause of the condition; (4) if case identification leads to improvement of workplace conditions, prevention of further claims should occur, thus benefiting both employee and employer; and (5) if these data are used for surveillance purposes, technical improvements in the data management system (e.g., better coding procedures or computer systems) could occur that would benefit the management of the workers' compensation insurance system itself.

In summary, workers' compensation data represent an important source of surveillance data that can be used to monitor trends in the occurrence of selected occupational disorders[11] and to identify cases for follow-up action.

Biological Monitoring Data
In selected situations, employers and health care providers obtain samples for biological monitoring (i.e., blood, urine, or hair) from workers exposed to toxic substances.[12] Typically, analyses are performed by one or only a few laboratories in a state. Data from the laboratory can be collected by a government agency and analyzed to monitor trends in exposure to selected toxic substances. This approach has certain limitations: (1) biological assays exist for only a few substances; (2) quality control programs for these analyses are limited; (3) participation in biological monitoring programs is often limited to larger firms in which hazards are well controlled; and (4) within firms that participate in a biological monitoring program, individual workers may choose not to be tested.

Nevertheless, there are advantages to this approach: (1) each test (e.g., blood lead concentration) is a specific index of exposure to the toxic substance of interest; and (2) in states where commercial laboratories are required to report results to the state agency, data can be obtained widely and at low additional cost.

In summary, for certain substances (blood lead testing is by far the best example), biological monitoring test results can be a useful source of surveillance data.

National Health Surveys
Each year, the U.S. National Center for Health Statistics (NCHS) performs surveys of statistical samples of the U.S. population. Within each sample, a subset of employed persons can be identified. In each survey, health status data and occupational listing information are collected. The U.S. Health Interview Survey (HIS) is a questionnaire survey that currently contacts 50,000 households, involving 130,000 individuals. In 1988, a supplement was added to the HIS to collect detailed occupational health information.

The National Health and Nutrition Examination Survey (NHANES) utilizes both a questionnaire and detailed medical tests to obtain health status information on 30,000 to 40,000 individuals. In 1988, NIOSH collaborated with NCHS researchers to include tests in the NHANES III protocol that evaluate selected occupational disorders: lung disorders and neurotoxicity. Thus, such national surveys represent useful sources of surveillance data for occupational health.[13]

Exposure Surveillance Systems

Exposure surveillance can be performed using existing data or through the performance of worksite surveys.[14] Existing environmental data are most commonly developed as part of compliance inspections performed by the U.S. Department of Labor (either OSHA or MSHA). Direct surveys have been performed by NIOSH, the National Occupational Hazard Survey, the National Occupational Exposure Survey, and the National Occupational Exposure Survey on Mining. Each approach has important advantages in describing trends in exposure to hazards in the workplace.

CONCLUSION

In the United States, a variety of surveillance systems exist (or are under development) for the identification of cases of occupational illness or injury and in the monitoring of trends. These programs should not be conducted as isolated activities, but rather integrated into a comprehensive program designed to control workplace hazards and protect worker health. Surveillance is a useful *secondary* prevention tool; control of hazardous conditions and exposures should be given *primary* consideration in the workplace.

Notes
1. Halperin, W. E., J. Ratcliffe, T. M. Frazier et al. 1986. Medical screening in the workplace: proposed principles. *J Occup Med* 28:547–552.
2. Halperin, W. E., P. A. Schulte, and D. C. Greathouse, eds. 1986. Conference on medical screening and biological monitoring for the effects of exposure in the workplace. *J Occup Med*
3. Matte, T. D., L. Fine, T. J. Meinhardt, and E. L. Baker. 1990. Guidelines for medical screening in the workplace. *Occup Med: State of the Art Reviews* 5:439–456.
4. Rothstein, M. A. 1984. *Medical Screening of Workers*. Washington, D.C.: Bureau of National Affairs.
5. Chinski, A. 1990. Medical surveillance in the workplace: legal issues. *Occup Med: State of the Art Reviews* 5:457–468.
6. Freund, E., P. J. Seligman, T. L. Chorba, S. K. Satford, J. G. Drachman, and H. F. Hull. 1989. Mandatory reporting of occupational diseases by clinicians. *JAMA* 262:3041–3044.
7. Baker, E. L. 1989. Sentinel Event Notification System for Occupational Risks (SENSOR): the concept. *Am J Public Health* 79(Suppl):18–20.
8. National Academy of Science. 1987. *Counting Injuries and Illness in the Workplace: Proposals for a Better System*. Washington, D.C.: National Academy Press.

9. Melius, J. M., J. P. Sestito, and P. J. Seligman. 1989. Occupational disease surveillance with existing data sources. *Am J Pub Health* 79(Suppl):46–52.
10. Harrahan, L. P., and M. B. Moll. 1989. Injury surveillance. *Am J Pub Health* 79(Suppl):38–45.
11. Seligman, P. J., W. E. Halperin, R. J. Mullen, and T. M. Frazier. 1986. Occupational lead poisoning in Ohio: surveillance using worker's compensation data. *Am J Pub Health* 76:1299–1302.
12. Rosenberg, J., and D. Rempel. 1990. Biological monitoring. *Occup Med: State of the Art Reviews* 5:491–498.
13. Ehrenberg, R. L., and J. E. Sniezek. 1989. Development of a standard questionnaire for occupational health research. *Am J Pub Health* 79(Suppl):15–17.
14. Froines, J., D. Wegman, and E. Eisen. 1989. Hazard surveillance in occupational disease. *Am J Pub Health* 79(Suppl):26–31.

14

Epidemiologic Surveillance Following Disasters

Roger I. Glass and Eric K. Noji

Disasters are extraordinary natural or manmade catastrophes that destroy property, disrupt society, and cause significant morbidity and mortality, and which can therefore overwhelm the capacity of the affected population to function normally. Over the past two decades, natural disasters worldwide have killed more than 3 million people and adversely affected the lives of 800 million.[1] In recent years, more than 30 million refugees, primarily in Asia and Africa, have been displaced when fleeing violence, civil war, political unrest, or famine.[2] Due to the massive impact of disasters on human health, the United Nations General Assembly has declared the 1990s to be the International Decade of Natural Disaster Reduction, and has called for a global effort to reduce the impact of these untoward events.[3] If this effort is to succeed, it will require considerable involvement by epidemiologists to determine how such reductions can be achieved.

The term "disaster" covers a range of events that drastically alter our natural environment, from geologic activity (e.g., earthquakes and volcanic eruptions) or severe weather (e.g., droughts, floods, and hurricanes) to manmade calamities (e.g., fires, chemical accidents, or wars). They can occur at one moment in time (e.g., tornados, earthquakes) or continue for long periods (e.g., droughts, radiation accidents). Some can be predicted well in advance (e.g., floods, hurricanes), while others cannot (e.g., earthquakes). Some occur with great frequency (e.g., tornados, hurricanes) while others are extremely rare (e.g., reactor meltdown). Finally, some affect millions of people (e.g., famine, earthquakes) while others can affect relatively few (e.g., bridge collapse). The unifying feature of disasters is the catastrophic effect these events can have on those that have experienced them and on a society's ability to respond. The health impact will vary greatly, as will the population's needs to return the society to working order.[4] The epidemiologist can provide timely assessments of the health problems related to the disaster in order to assist in mounting an effective, appropriate relief response, and to prevent similar consequences from future disasters.[5]

OBJECTIVES

Epidemiologic surveillance after a disaster involves the rapid assessment of the distribution and determinants of disaster-related deaths, illnesses, and injuries in the population affected, with the aim of determining their most immediate problems and matching these with a planned and appropriate response.[4a] Epidemiologists play a vital role in developing reliable information on the health consequences of the disaster, conducting surveys and investigations where necessary, providing advice on health problems that may arise, establishing priorities for action, and in emphasizing that proper decision-making requires timely and appropriate information.[6] The ultimate goal of epidemiologic surveillance is to prevent or reduce the adverse health consequences of the disaster itself as well as to optimize the decision-making process associated with management of the relief effort. These epidemiologic objectives can be simply defined as the surveillance cycle; that is, the collection of data, analysis of data, and response to data.[7]

The need for disaster epidemiology was apparent in many early disaster relief operations. Managers and planners with no public health expertise and no reliable information on the health of the population struck by disaster were forced to mount major relief efforts. In the absence of an adequate field assessment, their response was often dictated by the relief and medical assistance made available by donors. This led to the arrival on the disaster scene of outdated or inappropriate drugs, medical and surgical teams without proper support, and relief programs that did not address immediate local needs. These problems were all compounded in the vacuum created by the disaster, including the lack of communication, transportation, local supplies and support, and a decision-making structure. Since these relief operations were often conducted under the watchful eye of the media, medical relief efforts were often pejoratively called "the second disaster."[8]

In recent years, epidemiologic techniques have been effectively introduced as a basic component in many disaster relief operations. Epidemiologists have been able to define quickly the nature and extent of the health problems, identify groups in the population at particular risk for adverse health events, optimize the relief response, monitor the effectiveness of the relief effort, and provide recommendations to decrease the consequences from future disasters.[9] The low mortality associated with recent disasters such as hurricanes Gilbert (1988) and Hugo (1989), the San Francisco earthquake (1990), and tornados in North America represent the success of programs of weather forecasting and warning, disaster preparedness, emergency medical response, public awareness, and aseismic building codes; some of these efforts likely resulted from knowledge gathered through epidemiologic studies conducted as a consequence of previous disasters.

SPECIAL CONSIDERATIONS FOR DISASTER EPIDEMIOLOGY

The basic principles of epidemiologic surveillance after disasters are no different from surveillance applied in other settings.[10] However, in practice, the timeframe is often reduced if not instantaneous, epidemiologic information is incomplete, decision-making is by nature hasty, the relief response may be massive, visibility can be extensive, and chaos is ubiquitous. The surveillance cycle must turn many times: first with rapid, cursory assessments of problems using the most rudimentary data collection techniques, followed by short-term assessments involving the establishment of simple but reliable sources of data, and then with ongoing surveillance to identify continuing problems and monitor the response to the interventions chosen. Finally, in the aftermath of a disaster, focused analytic surveys can be used to compare victims with survivors and learn what could be done to prevent the human toll of morbidity in subsequent disasters. The success of the epidemic investigation of a disaster can be measured directly by how rapidly data collected and analyzed can identify prevention strategies, and how effectively these strategies can then be implemented by decision makers to direct relief and decrease ongoing morbidity. This effort requires active coordination between the epidemiologist, who gathers the data and identifies the issues or strategies, and the decision maker, who must understand the data and strategies and implement the required policies. In the rapid evolution of a disaster relief program, major decisions regarding relief are made early on, hastily, and often irreversibly; thus, the need for reliable early data to assist in making these decisions is crucial. A decision maker who questions a proposed intervention or donation can also use his epidemiologic capability to provide an independent and rapid assessment of need.

Field surveillance methods vary by disaster setting and the personnel

and time available. Early field surveys must follow the KISS principle—Keep It Simple, Stupid—and address the essential, most basic
questions requiring immediate answers that will directly prevent loss of
life or injury. Subsequently, surveys can address issues such as the
availability of medical care, assessment of the need for specific interventions, and epidemic control (e.g., establishment of a rumor clearinghouse
to receive information on epidemics of disease and provide for their
timely investigation), each of which demands more careful investigation.
Surveillance must be sensitive to monitor the impact of relief on the
health problems of the population, and to determine whether the effort
is having a tangible impact on the population or if new strategies are
needed. Surveillance becomes an iterative, cyclical process in which
simple health outcomes are constantly monitored and interventions
continually assessed for efficacy.

The attention span for relief after most natural disasters is short, measuring weeks to months, whereas the consequences for the population
affected can measure years or decades.[11] The aim of relief must be to help
the population quickly return to their predisaster state while investing
relief money and aid in ways to ensure the greatest long-term effect.[12] In
the early phase of relief, basic needs of water, food, clothing, shelter, and
medical care must be met, after which the longer-term process of rebuild-
ing proceeds. Relief aid can often be squandered early on by overreacting
to minor problems when excitement is great, needs are extensive, and
scrutiny by the media is omnipresent.[13] Longer-term goals are often overlooked even though they are generally more difficult and costly to achieve
and their impact can be longer lasting. Epidemiologic assessment, prioriti-
zation of needs, and planning an appropriate response can have a major
beneficial effect on the ability of a community to return to normalcy in
both the short and the longer term.

A repeated observation from many recent disasters is that the health
consequences of these events fall most heavily on people living in developing countries.[14] For example, earthquakes measuring 6–7 on the Richter
Scale led to massive loss of life in Peru (1970), Nicaragua (1972), Guate-
mala (1976), Tangshan, China (1976), and Armenia (1988), whereas quakes
of similar magnitude in California were associated with few health consequences despite considerable loss of property. Clearly, industrialized
countries are buffered from disasters by their ability to forecast severe
storms, enforce strict codes for aseismic and fireproof construction, utilize
communication networks to broadcast disaster warnings and alerts, provide emergency medical services, and engage in contingency planning to
prepare the population and public institutions for possible disasters. In
developing countries, such measures are either not available or have not

been implemented, and the populations thus remain more vulnerable to adverse health consequences from natural disasters.

EPIDEMIOLOGIC ISSUES OF DISASTER SURVEILLANCE

Famine Relief

In 1957, Sayler and Gordon, in one of the earliest reviews of the role of epidemiologic assessment after natural disasters, compared disasters to epidemics and suggested that they could be described in classic epidemiologic terms of time, place, and person.[15] This observation was similar to our change in thinking about accidents, which are no longer felt to be random events but have been renamed unintentional injuries subject to epidemiologic scrutiny. This concept was applied in the late 1960s to assist the massive international relief operation mounted to respond to famine conditions associated with the Nigerian civil war.[6] Epidemiologists developed new survey tools and survey methods to rapidly assess the nutritional status of large displaced populations so that relief could be targeted to those groups in greatest need. Subsequently, surveillance was critical to monitor the nutritional status of the population in response to the quantity and types of foods delivered. Rapid epidemiologic assessment proved invaluable to optimize food distribution practices in the face of rapidly changing conditions of health and relief. Since then, nutritional surveillance has become a routine part of relief work in famine areas and in refugee populations and is essential to rationalizing problems of food distribution.

Epidemic Control: A Rumor Clearinghouse

Epidemiologists have subsequently become involved in other aspects of postdisaster assessment. The Biblical fear of epidemic disease following disasters led many decision makers to enlist epidemiologists to investigate rumors of epidemics that were frequently reported. For example, following disasters in developing countries, any disruption of the water supply or sewage treatment was usually accompanied by rumors of outbreaks of cholera or typhoid. Such rumors may well have reflected psychological fears and anxieties about a disastrous event rather than the true perception of an imminent problem. Such epidemics are uncommon in the wake of natural disasters but can occur in settings such as refugee camps, where large populations of displaced persons are crowded together and share unsanitary conditions or contaminated water.[16] Nonetheless, a clearing-house can serve the important function of monitoring such rumors as they arise, investigating those that have merit in a timely fashion, dispelling those that are obviously false, and informing the public of hazards where a response is required. This concept has been helpful not only in developing countries but also in disasters occurring in urban settings of industrialized countries.

Surveillance of Preventable Deaths, Illnesses, and Injuries

The health problems associated with major disasters are usually more extensive than fears of epidemic diseases alone but are often measured in counts of people who died, were severely injured, or became ill. The epidemiologist must identify the most severe health consequences that can still be prevented by active, well-targeted interventions, and develop priorities to address them for the decision makers. These priorities likely differ for each disaster, challenging the epidemiologist to arrive rapidly with an appropriate plan. For example, because most deaths from earth-quakes occur during the initial impact, the prevention of subsequent mor-tality and severe injury requires early treatment of the injured or rapid extraction of those entrapped in collapsed buildings.[17] At the same time, attention must be given to earthquake-associated destruction of shelter, food and water supplies, roads and communication networks, and prob-lems of access to health care so that the survivors can be spared from subsequent health problems.[18] Since everyone in the disaster area will feel needs and experience loss, the challenge of the early assessment is to decide which needs and affected areas will most benefit from early inter-vention, preventing the greatest loss of life or most severe morbidity.

As an example, the usefulness of rapid epidemiologic surveillance to target a relief effort involving deaths, injuries, and often severe illness was demonstrated in 1979 when 30,000 Cambodians arrived as refugees in Thailand.[19] Escaping from the war, this group arrived in the Thai camps exhausted from fighting, short of food, injured, and heavily infected with malaria. Their high mortality was visible to the world when the interna-tional media reported that dead bodies were collected each morning for burial. A massive international relief operation was begun, but no informa-tion was available early on to determine whether relief efforts should be targeted to children or adults, or to problems of malnutrition, immuniza-tion, treatment of war injuries, or control of malaria and other epidemic diseases. The immediate aim of surveillance was to identify preventable causes of death immediately and to decide on the first priorities for relief.

The second aim of surveillance was to monitor mortality and morbidity to ascertain whether the relief effort was effective. In the absence of epidemiologic data, many media representatives described the refugees as living in "death camps," and associated this condition with a relief effort that was failing by not immediately preventing deaths.

Epidemiologic surveillance rapidly provided data on the rates of death, identified malaria as the principal cause of death and serious hospitalization, and led to specific strategies for the aggressive treatment of cerebral malaria, the primary cause of death. The swift decline in mortality during the first weeks of the effort was directly linked to a relief effort that had correctly targeted prevention issues. The collection of simple data on the daily number and presumed cause of deaths and admissions to the hospital, use of basic field surveys targeted to the specific questions of relief, and preparation of a brief weekly surveillance report made the relief effort responsive to the priority of health needs in the camp and provided reliable information both for donor organizations and the press. The use of epidemiologic teams to collect data, identify priorities, and monitor the effectiveness of the relief effort has become an integral part of many international relief and assistance groups.[9, 19]

Surveillance of Health Care Needs

In disasters associated with substantial numbers of victims with severe injuries (e.g., explosions, tornados) or illnesses (e.g., nuclear accidents, epidemics), the ability to prevent death or decrease severe morbidity will depend upon the provision of timely and adequate medical care, or to the triaging of victims to centers where such care is available.[20, 21] Rapid surveys of the number of victims needing special attention and the nature of the injuries or illnesses will have a direct impact on the response that can be mounted. Again, identifying the need for and monitoring the effect of the intervention are important epidemiologic functions.

Surveys to Avoid Unnecessary Interventions

After disasters, many agencies and donors offer supplies, equipment, and personnel for relief that are not always required. For example, the delivery of unnecessary, outdated, or unlabeled drugs to affected areas has been documented repeatedly following past disasters and is detrimental to the relief effort, causing a diversion of personnel to identify relevant supplies from a mass of unnecessary material.[22] Vaccines for cholera and typhoid fever have never been needed or effectively used following a disaster but are repeatedly offered, placing politicians and local personnel in the uncomfortable but correct position of saying "no." Disasters also often prompt an altruistic urge among health professionals. For example, no fewer than 30,000 physicians and nurses from the United States, Europe, Latin America, and Asia volunteered to work with Cambodian refugees in 1979–1980. The needs were limited in numbers, people with special skills and experience were required, and the efforts to select proper personnel were often difficult. Depending upon the pressures perceived by decision makers, the epidemiologists can often conduct surveys to assess whether interventions being volunteered by donors with significant political influence are in fact required.

Analytic Epidemiology: Prevention of Health Consequences from Future Disasters

In some disasters such as earthquakes, tornados, or hurricanes, a majority of deaths or severe injuries occur at the moment of the disaster itself. For each of these disasters, prevention strategies are often recommended that have never been subject to epidemiologic scrutiny. In recent years, epidemiologists have focused on assessing what strategies work best to prevent such disaster-related morbidity.[23] The questions raised follow a case-control design: Why did some people die (cases) while their neighbors, family members, or others survived (controls)? Risk factors for survival can range from prior knowledge and heeding of disaster warnings (e.g., tornado alerts), taking evasive action (e.g., seeking shelter in a stairwell), and availability of emergency medical care, to structural issues such as the building materials and codes adhered to for housing in an earthquake-prone area. Such analyses after earthquakes and tornados have each yielded new information that has altered traditional thinking on the prevention of disaster-related mortality. For example, in the Wichita Falls tornado in 1979, many people died while fleeing from the tornado's path in vehicles, a recommendation promoted by the weather service at that time.[24] An epidemiologic analysis determined that people who were caught in motor vehicles or motor homes had a 10- to 80-fold greater risk of death or severe injury than those who took shelter at home. Moreover, no severe injuries occurred among people who took shelter in basements or designated shelters in large public buildings. National advisories for the prevention of injury in tornados have been changed based upon these findings. Similarly, earthquake-related deaths are directly linked to construction practices, confirming the need for aseismic building codes, and to behavioral practices of fleeing buildings at the time of preshocks of earthquakes. However, even in developing countries, simple construction methods are available that have been epidemiologically associated with protection from the destructive forces of earthquakes. More analytic studies such as these are needed to test conventional warnings and advisories.

Anniversary Analysis of Relief Efforts

The long-term health consequences of disasters have never been properly assessed. No evaluations have been made five or ten years following a major disaster to determine whether changes in epidemiologic or relief practices, redirection of relief funds to longer-term goals, or changes in behavior or building patterns have had any long-term effect on a community's long-term response to disaster. Nonetheless, many communities that have experienced disaster are more concerned about preparedness efforts in the future.

CONCLUSIONS

The epidemiologist involved in disaster assessment faces a number of specific problems related to the political environment and rapidly changing health profile, needs, and opportunities to intervene. Data must be collected rapidly under highly adverse conditions. Epidemiologic information must be applied to a decision-making process since it can influence determining relief supplies, equipment, and personnel needed to respond effectively. Standardized procedures for collecting data in disasters need to be developed that can be linked to operational decisions and actions.

A variety of epidemiologic methods has been demonstrated to be of value before, during, and after disasters. Before the disaster, energies must be focused on delineating the populations at risk, and on assessing the level of emergency preparedness, the flexibility of existing surveillance systems, and the training of personnel. During impact, the health care needs of the affected population and the needs for emergency services have to be assessed quickly with the goal of preventing avoidable death, injury, or illness. In the post-impact phase, continuous monitoring and surveillance of the health problems faced by the population are required, as well as information on the effectiveness of relief interventions. After the disaster, epidemiologic methods can be used to evaluate in an iterative fashion the effectiveness of each health intervention program. Incorporation of epidemiologic surveillance and disaster management can dramatically reduce the health consequences of these catastrophic events on the affected population.

Notes
1. National Research Council. 1987. *Confronting Natural Disasters: An International Decade for Natural Disaster Reduction*. Washington, D.C.: National Academy Press.

2. Toole, M. J., and R. J. Waldman. 1990. Prevention of excess mortality in refugee and displaced populations in developing countries. *JAMA* 263: 3296–3302.

3. U.N. General Assembly. 18 October 1988. International Decade for Natural Disaster Reduction: Report of the Secretary-General. 43rd Session, agenda item 86, A/43/723.

4. Seaman, J. 1984. Epidemiology of natural disasters. *Contributions to Epidemiol and Biostat* M. A. Klingberg, ed., Basel, Switzerland: S. Karger 5:1–177.

4a. Guha-Sapir, D. 1991. Rapid assessment of health needs in mass emergencies: Review of current concepts and methods. *Wld Hlth Statist Quart* 44:171–181.

5. Binder, S., and L. M. Sanderson. 1987. The role of the epidemiologist in natural disasters. *Ann Emerg Med 16:1081–1084*.

6. Western, K. 1972. The epidemiology of natural and man-made disasters: the present state of the art. Ph.D. Thesis. London: London School of Hygiene and Tropical Medicine, University of London.

7. Foege, W. H. 1986. Public health aspects of disaster management. In J. M. Last, ed. *Public Health and Preventive Medicine*, 1879–1886. Norwalk, Conn.: Appleton-Century-Croft.

8. Lechat, M. F. 1990. Updates: the epidemiology of health effects of disasters. *Epid Rev* 12:192–197.

9. Editorial. 1990. Disaster epidemiology. *Lancet* 336:845–846.

10. Gregg, M. B., ed. 1986. *The Public Health Consequences of Disasters*. Atlanta, Ga.: U.S. Department of Health and Human Services.

11. Hagman, G. 1984. *Prevention Better than Cure*. Stockholm: Swedish Red Cross.

12. Cuny, F. 1983. *Disasters and Development*. Oxford: Oxford University Press.

13. Seaman, J. 1990. Disaster epidemiology: or why most international disaster relief is ineffective. *Injury* 21:5–8.

14. Wijkman, A., and L. Timberlake. 1984. *Natural Disasters: Acts of God or Acts of Man*. New York: Earthscan Paperback.

15. Sayler, L. F., and J. E. Gordon. 1957. The medical component of natural disasters. *Am J Med Sci* 234:342–362.

16. de Ville de Goyet, C., and J. L. Zeballos. 1988. Communicable diseases and epidemiological surveillance after sudden natural disasters. In Baskett, P., and R. Weller, eds. *Medicine for Disasters*, 252–269. London: Wright.

17. Glass, R. I., J. J. Urrutia, S. Sibony et al. 1977. Earthquake injuries related to housing in a Guatemalan village. *Science* 197:638–643.

18. Noji, E. K., G. D. Kelen, H. K. Armenian et al. 1990. The 1988 earthquake in Soviet Armenia: a case study. *Ann Emerg Med* 19:891–897.

19. Glass, R. I., P. Nieburg, W. Cates et al. 1980. Rapid assessment of health status and preventive medicine needs of newly arrived Kampuchean refugees, SaKaeo, Thailand. *Lancet* 1:868–872.

20. Safar, P. 1986. Resuscitation potentials in mass disasters. *Prehosp and Disaster Med* 2:34–47.

21. Waeckerle, J. F. 1991. Disaster planning and response. *NEJM* 324:815–821.

22. Autier, P., M. Ferir, A. Hairapetien et al. 1990. Drug supply in the aftermath of the 1988 Armenian earthquake. *Lancet* 335:1388–1390.
23. Noji, E. K., and K. T. Sivertson. 1987. Injury prevention in natural disasters: a theoretical framework. *Disasters* 11:290–296.
24. Glass, R. I., R. B. Craven, D. J. Bregman, B. J. Stoll, N. Horowitz, P. Kerndt, and J. Winkle. 1980. Injuries from the Wichita Falls tornado: implications for prevention. *Science* 207:734–738.

15

Pharmacosurveillance: Public Health Monitoring of Medication

Hugh H. Tilson

INTRODUCTION: WHAT IS PHARMACOSURVEILLANCE?

The field of pharmacoepidemiology devotes the tools, expertise, energies, and philosophies of epidemiology to the public health issues raised by the use of medications. All pharmacologic agents, no matter how elegant the underlying science and how targeted the therapeutic intervention, have effects beyond those immediately desired. Call them side effects, adverse events, drug reactions, toxicity, or by another name, adverse drug experiences (ADEs) must always be taken into account when choosing to introduce a pharmacologic intervention into a disease process, and even more so when using medication for prevention.

At the level of individual medical practice (the micropolicy level), the decision-making process that leads to the choice to use medication, and then to the choice of the exact medication, involves a complex epidemiologic and medical logic—balancing everything the physician knows about the likely benefit of the agent against what is known about its likely or possible risks. In this regard, as with other targets of epidemiologic monitoring, this field is one that offers endless challenges to the monitoring capacities of society, enabling the prescriber and the patient to know what they need to know to make an enlightened decision. To do these important social jobs, the tools of epidemiology provide a vital complement to those of experimental and clinical pharmacology. Epidemiologic intelligence or surveillance approaches are needed to detect and assemble for action the important signals of potential problems from a medicine's use; the structured observational epidemiologic study, cohort or case-control, is needed to quantitate such signals. By extension, a similar epidemiologic basis is needed at the population, or macropolicy, level. Society needs information concerning the risk-to-benefit ratio of each of the agents available for therapeutic choice. Considering the differences in safety profiles can become the driving force in formulary committee decisions. At the national level, an ongoing process is needed to modify the conditions of approval to market (e.g., change the approved label to reflect evolving information) and, in extreme circumstances, to withdraw or recall a product. At the international level, a coordination of activities is needed to assure that we get the most accurate, understandable, powerful information—without duplicating efforts.

THE NEED FOR PHARMACOEPIDEMIOLOGY: LIMITS OF KNOWLEDGE AT THE TIME OF NEW DRUG APPROVAL

In our modern society as never before, the process of drug development is elegant, thorough, and careful. The development of new drugs is governed by complex national and international regulatory processes, and addressed through equally complex and rigorous scientific approaches. A public outcry for closer drug regulation arose following the thalidomide disaster, in which a horrible side effect—the congenital defect, phocomelia—occurred in association with use of a mild sedative and hypnotic. Thousands of babies were born with diminished and/or deformed limbs before our social monitoring systems detected the problem.[1] The result around the world was tighter and more specific governmental monitoring of the process of drug development. In the United States, this was reflected by the revision of the Food, Drug and Cosmetics Act to require substantial proof of safety and efficacy under the New Drug Application (NDA) clauses.[2] Requiring proof of efficacy (by subsequent guidelines in two "well-controlled clinical trials"), this legislation and the responsible attitude of academia and industry accompanying it have resulted in the launch of an era in which the randomized, blinded, controlled clinical trial has become the "gold standard," and in which the science of drug development has reached a sophistication never before equalled.

However, in the face of this blossoming good science, two other realities have loomed large. First, the costs of conducting such elegant clinical research have skyrocketed. It is currently estimated that the average new drug costs in excess of $200 million from the bench to the market.[3] Thus, economic pressures are enormous to streamline the research process to its irreducible minimum compatible with such good science. The result is highly targeted, carefully calculated studies directed at highly focused endpoints. It is not unusual, therefore, that a new drug will be marketed with experience in 2,000 patients or less. The implications for the public's health relating to drug-associated toxicities are substantial. Most commonly occurring side effects will be well-known—the occasional headache, nausea, rash, or other minor annoyance as an accompanying effect of medication.[4] Certainly, commonly occurring and potentially dangerous side effects will also be known and, if a substantial threat to health, may have resulted in the termination of the clinical trials program and the failure of that drug to reach the market. And, fortunately, still, once drugs reach this level of sophisticated development, they are "remarkably nontoxic"—with very few "surprises" occurring subsequently.[5] However, surprises such as serious, unexpected, or even potentially fatal, although infrequent side effects—those occurring, for example, in less than 1 out of every 10,000 therapies—could not possibly be known in the course of a drug development program with only 2,000 patients involved. This has been the case in the years since the thalidomide disaster of the early 1960s with only a handful of major therapeutic agents. However, the morbidity and mortality associated with these drug-induced epidemics have been substantial. In each case, the outcome was severe; the need for a public health–oriented drug-induced side effects safety monitoring program was equally clear: to determine the existence of such side effects as clearly as possible and as rapidly as possible, in order to protect society against major unforeseen and wholly unpredictable side effects of new medicines.

Second, there is another substantial reason why not everything can be known about a new drug's safety at the time it is marketed. Part of the focus of the clinical trials program is to restrict the complexity of the patients tested, the endpoints procured, and the duration of therapy and monitoring. Thus, not included in drug testing will be many persons who are likely eventually to receive new medicines—the chronically and severely ill, the very young and the very old, the woman in the childbearing years, the fetus in utero.

Such complex patients and circumstances pose complex problems for the methodologist; it often will be viewed as impractical or prohibitively expensive to test new drugs in such groups; it would generally be considered unethical in some cases, as in experimentation on the fetus or the newborn; and usually it is impractical to monitor many years of chronic therapy or for many years beyond the initial therapy to determine the effects of long latency. Following their marketing, however, new medicines will be used in these populations, and useful or potentially useful and/or unintended exposures will occur as a result (e.g., women taking a new medicine may become pregnant). Learning from this "natural experiment" becomes a critical opportunity—in this area as for many others in this book—for the nonexperimental, observational tools of epidemiology.

PHARMACOSURVEILLANCE: EPIDEMIOLOGIC INTELLIGENCE APPLIED TO PHARMACEUTICALS

Given the limitations of pre-approval science, it is not difficult to understand why the process of drug regulation and approval is such a difficult one. One is always confronted with the dilemma that there are limits to the extent to which one can be certain of safety from a sample which is both limited in number and in representativeness and comprehensiveness. Yet, there are limits to the number of persons one can require to have included in the program of pre-approval drug testing; the duration of such tests; and the duration of follow-up. Thus, having been monitored in perhaps as few as 2,000 persons altogether, for as brief a period as 12 months or less, the needed new medicines are approved for marketing by regulatory authorities around the world.

When a new drug is approved, the technical act is the approval of an application for a new drug (NDA, or its counterparts worldwide) to permit the manufacturer to market it, while requiring the manufacturer to draw parameters around the claims of efficacy and the warnings regarding its safety. However, recognizing that individual patient circumstances differ widely, that experience evolves through incremental learning and trial and error, and—most fundamental for this discussion—that it is unreasonable for us to expect to know everything at the time a new drug is approved, the manufacturer's limitations and stipulations do not restrict the latitude of prescribing physicians to use medicines in ways that they find them to be well-suited. Thus, a period of sociomedical experimentation is launched in which many times more persons will be treated—even in the first few months following approval—than were treated during the entire clinical trials program, and the conditions of their treatment will differ from those for which there is documented experimental evidence.

Thus, it is critical that we have a system of monitoring that will enable us to learn from this experience. In the United States, this is the spontaneous voluntary adverse reactions reports monitoring system, which applies the basic principles of epidemiologic intelligence and reportable disease disciplines from other areas in public health to the issues relating to experience with medications. In contrast with communicable disease surveillance, physicians are asked to monitor their patients' experiences with medicines, to recognize and diagnose drug-associated adverse events, and report them *voluntarily* either to the manufacturer or directly to the regulatory authority. The standard form for reporting adverse reactions is the Food and Drug Administration's Form FDA 1639 (see Figure 15-1). The FDA, in communication with physicians on an ongoing basis through its "FDA Drug Bulletin," regularly distributes fresh copies of FDA 1639 and urges physicians to report directly.

In the United States, however, an essential element of the spontaneous reporting system is the pharmaceutical manufacturer. Over 85 percent of all spontaneous adverse reactions reports in the United States enter this system through some kind of interaction with the manufacturer. Several circumstances have contributed to this. Pharmaceuticals are "detailed" by professional pharmaceutical manufacturers' representatives in physicians' offices. As part of this educational endeavor, dialogue regarding the physicians' experiences will doubtless evolve; and if a sales representative becomes aware that there has been an adverse experience in the practice of the physician, she or he is therefore "on notice" and the company, having been notified, will institute procedures to define the problem and further report it to the FDA.[6] Unlike the practitioner, the manufacturer is obligated under federal regulation to report all such experiences to the FDA.

A second major source of adverse experience complaints to industry is the evolving sector of drug information. In the community, this is embodied by the drug information pharmacist, frequently found in major teaching institutions making rounds with house staff and available to answer medication-associated questions for all professionals. An adverse experience detected on rounds or called to the attention of the drug information pharmacist may become the subject of an official report. More likely, it will be the subject of an informal inquiry to the manufacturer. In turn, the industry over the past decade has developed programs of drug information in order to respond to these kinds of inquiries. If an inquiry involves an adverse drug experience, the company is once again "on notice." Finally, direct inquiry and notification by practitioners, patients, or other intermediaries (e.g., a friend, a nurse, a pharmacist, an attorney) constitute the remainder of reports coming directly to the attention of the manufacturer.

Similar systems exist in Europe, Australia, and Japan, and are increasingly being formalized throughout the world wherever medications are used. Indeed, the World Health Organization (WHO) has a spontaneous adverse reactions reports registry with 27 national centers cooperatively participating, that submit approximately 60,000 reports per year.

Sampling, as the systems do, from the entire "universe" of practice experience, they have a very powerful denominator—namely, all of the

DEPARTMENT OF HEALTH AND HUMAN SERVICES PUBLIC HEALTH SERVICE FOOD AND DRUG ADMINISTRATION (HFN-730) ROCKVILLE, MD 20857 **ADVERSE REACTION REPORT** **(Drugs and Biologics)**	Form Approved: OMB No. 0910-0230.
	FDA CONTROL NO.
	ACCESSION NO.

I. REACTION INFORMATION

1. PATIENT IDANITIALS (In Confidence)	2. AGE YRS.	3. SEX	4.-6. REACTION ONSET			8.-12. CHECK ALL APPROPRIATE:
			MO.	DA.	YR.	

7. DESCRIBE REACTION(S)

☐ PATIENT DIED

☐ REACTION TREATED WITH Rx DRUG

☐ RESULTED IN, OR PROLONGED, INPATIENT HOSPITALIZATION

☐ RESULTED IN PERMANENT DISABILITY

13. RELEVANT TESTS/LABORATORY DATA

☐ NONE OF THE ABOVE

II. SUSPECT DRUG(S) INFORMATION

14. SUSPECT DRUG(S) (Give manufacturer and lot no. for vaccines/biologics)	20. DID REACTION ABATE AFTER STOPPING DRUG?
15. DAILY DOSE — 16 ROUTE OF ADMINISTRATION	☐ YES ☐ NO ☐ NA
17. INDICATION(S) FOR USE	21. DID REACTION REAPPEAR AFTER REINTRODUCTION?
18. DATES OF ADMINISTRATION (From/To) — 19 DURATION OF ADMINISTRATION	☐ YES ☐ NO ☐ NA

III. CONCOMITANT DRUGS AND HISTORY

22. CONCOMITANT DRUGS AND DATES OF ADMINISTRATION (Exclude those used to treat reaction)

23. OTHER RELEVANT HISTORY (e.g. diagnoses, allergies, pregnancy with LMP, etc.)

IV. ONLY FOR REPORTS SUBMITTED BY MANUFACTURER	V. INITIAL REPORTER (In confidence)
24. NAME AND ADDRESS OF MANUFACTURER (Include Zip Code)	26.-26a. NAME AND ADDRESS OF REPORTER (Include Zip Code)
24a. IND/NDA. NO. FOR SUSPECT DRUG — 24b MFR. CONTROL NO.	26b. TELEPHONE NO. (Include area code)
24c. DATE RECEIVED BY MANUFACTURER — 24d. REPORT SOURCE (Check all that apply) ☐ FOREIGN ☐ STUDY ☐ LITERATURE ☐ HEALTH PROFESSIONAL ☐ CONSUMER	26c. HAVE YOU ALSO REPORTED THIS REACTION TO THE MANUFACTURER? ☐ YES ☐ NO
25 15 DAY REPORT? ☐ YES ☐ NO — 25a REPORT TYPE ☐ INITIAL ☐ FOLLOWUP	26d. ARE YOU A HEALTH PROFESSIONAL? ☐ YES ☐ NO
NOTE: Required of manufacturers by 21 CFR 314.80	Submission of a report does not necessarily constitute an admission that the drug caused the adverse reaction.

FORM FDA 1639 (7 86)   PREVIOUS EDITION MAY BE USED

FIGURE 15-1.   The FDA adverse reaction report.

prescriptions for an entire nation—from which to generate the "signals" of an adverse experience. On the other hand, relying as they also do upon voluntary reporting from a busy clinician, and involving as they do the rather complex arena of clinical pharmacology, the systems have substantial limitations. In order to be reported, an adverse experience must come to the level of recognition (e.g., result in a medical visit for a symptom or sign in the patient); it must be recognized and acknowledged as important; it must somehow be intuitively linked to the medication exposure that preceded it; then it must occasion the report.[7] However, in a recent survey of physicians in Maryland, Dr. Audrey Rogers[8] reported that only 37 percent said that they had seen a moderate or serious adverse drug reaction in their practice during the preceding year (although, of course, such adverse experiences must be occurring in every practice!). Of those who had seen them, only 5 percent reported them. Reasons for not reporting ranged from considering them unimportant; assuming that they were already "known"; and not knowing that there was a system into which they should be reported . . . a distressing 43 percent!

INTERNATIONAL COORDINATION

Geographic considerations are not unimportant to monitoring medication-associated adverse experiences, though they do differ from those in other surveillance applications. In general, the use of medications tends to be nation-specific, and each nation has its own independent drug approval processes. Therefore, medicines may be approved in one but not in an adjacent nation. While some nations do tend to be "earlier" approvers and others later, for any individual medication the time in sequence for approval will be unique—especially when there are considerations of the nations either in which the drug was initially developed or in which the company resides that will eventually market it internationally. Epidemiologic monitoring of medication-associated side effects likewise differs widely from nation to nation, with varying definitions of what is reportable and how it is to be reported, and distinct relationships among industry, practice, academia, and government. Thus, for example, while 85 percent of all spontaneous reports surfacing in the U.S. system are submitted by manufacturers, in the United Kingdom 85 percent are reported directly by practitioners to the Committee on Safety of Medicines using a very simplified report form, the "Yellow Card".[9] The reporting rates from practicing physicians also differ dramatically from nation to nation.[10] In an effort to try to rationalize this crazy quilt of reporting requirements, the Council on International Organizations for the Medical Sciences (CIOMS) has convened an international Adverse Drug Reaction (ADR) working group. As a result of its first several years of deliberations, the CIOMS group created a demonstration project in which the seven participating nations agreed to a single set of definitions regarding seriousness, unexpectedness, and the reportability of serious, unexpected adverse experiences. Given common definitions, the group also agreed on a single, standardized international form by which multinational pharmaceutical houses might report ADRs from outside the nation to that nation's regulatory authority (the so-called CIOMS form; see Figure 15-2).[11] This working group continues to explore other areas for better-coordinated international safety reporting.

The fundamental principle applicable to all multinational surveillance systems is that individual national experiences will vary and need to be seen as unique, yet must be analyzed in association with the experiences of all other nations that might participate in a multinational surveillance effort. To ignore the experiences of the various monitoring nations is to diminish the denominator and with it the power of the sentinel. However, to simply merge them is to oversimplify a very complicated and diverse reporting structure with different reporters reporting in different ways to different recipients at different rates. Multinational comparisons have been most useful when a "signal" was generated in one but not another nation. To help understand what else might be going on in the sentinel nation that might account for a difference in the signal, several considerations are imperative. These range from simple chance occurrence in one but not another nation; to a difference in reporting rates that is derivative of the difference in monitoring approaches; to a true difference that is a result of differences in medical treatments or practice, of other medications also on the market, or, even rarely, of ethnic differences.[12] This becomes particularly complex when one nation takes aggressive regulatory action; for example, recalls and/or bans from sale a product for which there are not significant safety signals in another country. In the past, what may have been unthinkable has now in the 1990s become a practical, international, regulatory reality: Regulators from several nations are speaking with each other and attempting to reconcile differing points of view; regardless, a regulatory action in one country will not inexorably lead to parallel regulatory actions in all countries, as, for example, with the Fenoterol debate and Pacific Island patients.[13a, 13b]

OTHER SOURCES OF EPIDEMIOLOGIC INTELLIGENCE

The mainstay of epidemiologic intelligence relating to pharmaceuticals is the spontaneous voluntary adverse reactions report, with individual

CIOMS FORM

SUSPECT ADVERSE REACTION REPORT

I. REACTION INFORMATION

1 PATIENT INITIALS (first, last)	1a COUNTRY	2 DATE OF BIRTH Day Month Year	2a AGE Years	3 SEX	4 6 REACTION ONSET Day Month Year	8-12 CHECK ALL APPROPRIATE TO ADVERSE REACTION

7 - 13 DESCRIBE REACTION(S) (including relevant tests/lab data)

- PATIENT DIED
- INVOLVED OR PROLONGED INPATIENT HOSPITALISATION
- INVOLVED PERSISTENCE OR SIGNIFICANT DISABILITY OR INCAPACITY
- LIFE THREATENING

II. SUSPECT DRUG(S) INFORMATION

14 SUSPECT DRUG(S) (include generic name)		20 DID REACTION ABATE AFTER STOPPING DRUG? ☐ YES ☐ NO ☐ NA
15 DAILY DOSES	16 ROUTE(S) OF ADMINISTRATION	21. DID REACTION REAPPEAR AFTER REINTRODUCTION? ☐ YES ☐ NO ☐ NA
17 INDICATION(S) FOR USE		
18 THERAPY DATES (from/to)	19 THERAPY DURATION	

III. CONCOMITANT DRUG(S) AND HISTORY

22. CONCOMITANT DRUG(S) AND DATES OF ADMINISTRATION (exclude those used to treat reaction)

23. OTHER RELEVANT HISTORY (e.g. diagnostics, allergies, pregnancy with last month of period, etc.)

IV. MANUFACTURER INFORMATION

24a. NAME AND ADDRESS OF MANUFACTURER	
	24b. MFR CONTROL NO
24c DATE RECEIVED BY MANUFACTURER	24d REPORT SOURCE ☐ STUDY ☐ LITERATURE ☐ HEALTH PROFESSIONAL
DATE OF THIS REPORT	25a REPORT TYPE ☐ INITIAL ☐ FOLLOWUP

FIGURE 15-2.   The CIOMS form.

national systems being complemented by similar surveillance worldwide. However, the pharmacosurveillance officer also has available a series of other sources of intelligence information: continuing clinical drug trials, official and unofficial registry reports, and the world's published literature.

Continuing Clinical Studies

Following the approval of a new drug for marketing, the process of drug development has certainly not been completed; indeed, it has really only just begun for many drugs. Further clinical testing, undertaken against other therapeutic agents, to refine dose and regimen, and to target new uses—not to mention to further demonstrate usefulness—is the rule, not the exception, and clinical trials will also be conducted in other countries where the product has not yet been marketed. From all of these clinical studies, continued accumulation of adverse experience databases, particularly with a "proper" denominator, is the rule. And while true meta-analysis is quite inappropriate to compare the widely disparate experimental approaches, settings, and questions, in the crudest sense the world receives an accumulated denominator (persons registered in clinical trials) and its appropriate accumulated numerator (all of the occurrences of important serious adverse events in all clinical trials combined). Because the experimental setting is one in which the closest reasonable monitoring is in effect—that is, by professionals with the greatest possible interest in clinical pharmacology—it is the most likely to have the most accurate detection and attribution. Thus, the continuing contribution of drug development to surveillance activities must not be underestimated, albeit limited primarily by the intensive restraints upon clinical trial size and scope already discussed.

Registries

Many nations make their official spontaneous voluntary adverse reactions reports registries available to epidemiologic surveillance officers in other countries, including to the manufacturer; for example, the United States under the Freedom of Information Act, or the United Kingdom in its Anonymized Single Patient Profile (ASPP) system. Others actually publish their entire adverse experience database on a regular periodic basis and, with just reason, will permit specific (though limited) inquiries regarding specific cases (e.g., Sweden, Australia). The largest and most ambitious of these efforts are those of the World Health Organization (WHO) Collaborating Center in Uppsala, Sweden.[14] Efforts are underway to improve timeliness (in the past these data have lagged sorely) and availability (in the past, data have not been generally available to the surveillance community). Registries also exist of serious side effects in which regular, routine medication histories are obtained and in which, therefore, "simultaneous mini-case control studies" can be conducted (e.g., serious cutaneous adverse reactions registries, drug-induced ocular or dermatologic side effects registries, etc.). Perhaps the most widely known and used of these are the birth defects registries.

Published Literature

The published literature represents a powerful resource for the dissemination of important, new clinical pharmacologic information, including the broadcast of possible ADR signals. The clinical case report, found in most clinical journals, may be the first major "signal" of an important side effect. In fact, a favorite turn of phrase of persons publishing their favorite case is "this is the first reported case of X in association with Y . . . ." Epidemiologic intelligence officers accumulate all such published cases and analyze them in the same way that they analyze reports spontaneously from the field. Indeed, in the United States, the Food and Drug Administration regulations require that all adverse experiences in the published literature be monitored and the important ones reported by manufacturers under guidelines similar to those for spontaneous reports.[15] Guidelines for such literature monitoring and reporting at the international level are also under discussion by the continuing CIOMS Drug Safety Work Group.

THE STRUCTURED EPIDEMIOLOGIC STUDY

A rapidly evolving major contribution of the field of epidemiology to drug safety monitoring is the structured epidemiologic observational (nonexperimental) study of drug-disease associations, using case-control and cohort/ follow-up methods. Such studies are, more and more, being launched at the same time that the drug is first launched into the marketplace to complement, extend, and "firm up" the findings of epidemiologic intelligence with more clearly and completely defined populations (denominators: perhaps 10,000 to 20,000 persons) with closer and more complete event monitoring (the numerator). Detailed methodologic discussions of such research approaches are beyond the scope of a chapter on surveillance. Suffice it to say, close monitoring of large cohorts can materially strengthen the safety database upon which clinical and public health recommendations must be drawn.

MONITORING FOR WHAT?

All surveillance systems must have a purpose: the earliest possible/practicable detection of important problems that warrant some form of social action. In the case of medications monitoring, this translates into the frame of reference of prescription medicines. At its extreme, a medication may be found to have a rare but unacceptable toxicity which will result in its removal from the market. The earlier this is detected and the faster regulatory action is initiated, the better for all concerned. In this corner of commercial epidemiology—perhaps unlike other sectors where there is a broader separation between commerce and health—medications are seen by their manufacturers as part of the health care enterprise, and pharmaceutical companies see themselves as part of health care. Therefore, just as no department of surgery would wish to advance a surgical procedure once it was determined to be hazardous, no matter how great the pride in innovation and technology, so too, no pharmaceutical firm would wish to market a substance that was unacceptably hazardous. Determining, however, what is acceptable involves sometimes heroic epidemiologic leaps of faith—reasoning from "signals" of variable strength and quality and assessing all other options for intervention.

However, none of the actors involved in the decision would take removal from the market lightly. Medications are developed and marketed to relieve human suffering. Even the most apparently "copy cat" agents will have unique features, and patients who have a unique responsiveness to them. Based on the best estimate that the average drug development process costs in excess of $200 million for every new entity to reach the marketplace, the recall of such a product results in enormous losses—potentially catastrophic for an individual drug developer and terribly costly for a cost-conscious sector. Thus, such a major decision balances acceptable risk versus necessary social benefit and is a complicated one indeed. However, regardless of these considerations, most of the products of epidemiologic monitoring of medication safety are less dramatic. The major objective is to help to optimize prescription/medication practices by providing better clarity and quantitation to the safety warnings to enable the prescriber to make more balanced recommendations for therapy against alternative medications and/or interventions—in short, to optimize therapeutic decision-making.

A series of tools represent the methods at the disposal of the sector to translate risk messages into therapeutic decision-making. The "final common pathway" for medication safety messages tends to be the learned intermediary, the prescriber, in contrast to many other surveillance systems. And the common denominator information tool for that prescriber is the official product label/"package insert." Published in the *Physicians Desk Reference (PDR)* and printed on an insert—often a very long, detailed, small-print official document—that accompanies every package of medication, the package insert is the subject of detailed negotiation with the regulatory agency. The negotiation of the wording of the insert aims to ensure that no claims are made regarding the product in excess of those that can be scientifically justified, and that no safety warning is omitted for which there is adequate reason to warn. The prescribing information also accompanies product promotional information officially distributed by the manufacturer. In the event of a new and important warning, the manufacturer may communicate directly with prescribers, such as in a "Dear Doctor" official notification of new and important safety information. And, at the broadest level, the published scientific literature and scientific symposium program are replete with descriptions of medication experience, further to fine-tune the physician's understanding of the balance of benefits to risks in individual agents and across therapeutic classes.

In other words, surveillance for signals of medicine-induced injury regularly and systematically results in a restructuring of the way medicine is practiced. As important events come to the attention of the signaling system, if the signal is strong and clear, if a good pharmacologic case for causality or possible causality can be made, and if it is important for practicing physicians, nurses, pharmacists (and the millions of other readers of the *PDR,* the second best-selling, nonfiction book after the Bible), new information gets fed into the product label (package insert) all the time. A recent report from the Government Accounting Office (GAO) on the safety of medicines reviewed package labels of 209 new products marketed during the period of the survey. In over half of these products, a "major" safety warning was added to the label following approval, a tribute to the effective and useful function of the surveillance mechanism.[16] An important corollary finding was that only six of these were removed from the market because the import of these side effects tipped the balance of risk-to-benefit such that the former outweighed the latter.

Like all public health surveillance, this system has as one of its motivations providing society protection against a major "epidemic" with the sensitive triggering of necessary—and sometimes quite aggressive—intervention mechanisms. In pharmacosurveillance, such findings might, conceivably, result in marketing withdrawal of a product.[17-21] For example, when suprofen (Suprol®) was marketed in 1986, sporadic reports were received of a syndrome involving severe flank pain in association with its use (though remarkably not associated with other visible nephrotoxicity). News of these signals, because of their severity and frequency, was transmitted to practicing physicians by the manufacturer in a "Dear Doctor" letter, which resulted in a deluge of yet further reports. Within a period of three months the manufacturer determined the extent and severity of the signal to be such as to warrant a voluntary market withdrawal.[22] A second classic example of the excellent use of signaling is the withdrawal of the antidepressant zimelidine (Zelmid®) from the market in Sweden on the basis of a cluster of reports of associated Guillain-Barré syndrome. Here the population expected rate was 2.5/100,000/yr; a maximum population exposure based on sales was 60,000 (which translated into 14,000 patient-years); and six to eight cases had been reported. There was, on its face, little doubt and thus little need for further study before necessary action![23]

WHAT'S WRONG WITH THIS PICTURE?

Not all that "beeps" is a true "signal," of course.

An attribute that differentiates surveillance of pharmaceuticals from the other surveillance activities addressed in this book is the issue of confounding by indication. People take medicines for a reason. Further-more, the reasons for the choice of any specific medication—"the indica-tion"—are many and complex. For example, once approved a medication may be used for any number of conditions that do not appear in the approved package labeling, or for which the efficacy of the agent has not been completely proven. Thus, no assumptions can be made when study-ing drug-disease associations about indication. If the reason for use isn't known or hasn't been stated, then, at very least, a caveat needs to be issued about any association. And at best, a specific survey is needed to understand the indication. The natural history of the disease being treated and its nonpharmacologic complications may easily be confused with unwanted side effects.

Most adverse effects of drugs are manifest by signs and symptoms that are not unique and/or pathognomonic for that drug or for a drug cause at all. A headache is a headache is a headache. Of course, if headache is also one of the "side effects" of the disease being treated, then differentiation of the disease effect from the drug effect in the individual may be difficult if not impossible. Since spontaneous reporting requires attribution (or at least an index of suspicion); attribution involves differentiation from the expected; and side effects may differ from expected effects only insofar as they are more frequent rather than clinically differentiated, it is often very difficult to recognize such events as side effects. Conversely, every-body wants to find a reason for things—particularly bad things. Therefore, when bad things happen to good people (my patients) I will tend to look for a reason, even when there isn't necessarily a reason. And, proximate cause logic being what it is, the fact that a medication was given shortly before a bad event occurred may become the reason—perhaps the only reason—for an attribution. Consider, for example, the situation with adverse outcomes of pregnancy. The world of pharmacoepidemiology is (and always must be) on the lookout for another thalidomide, which might cause an epidemic of a birth defect if taken during the first trimester (and to a lesser extent because of adverse impact upon gestation, during later trimesters) of pregnancy. On the other hand, birth defects occur in more than 3 percent of all pregnancies carried to term. Therefore, 3 percent of the time, in association with the use of the therapeutic agent under surveillance, pregnancies with a first trimester exposure will result in a birth defect. Since most congenital anomalies have no specific known "cause," such an outcome is not unlikely to become the object of a spontaneous voluntary adverse experience report by mis-attribution.

Issues of confounding by indication or chance association are particularly topical in today's environment—with AIDS and its complicating conditions becoming increasingly prevalent and rapidly changing before our eyes—often as a result of improved therapies themselves. Absent a well-charted natural history of disease, rare complications of that disease will begin to be noticed as people survive longer. Thus, survival and its complications will both be associated with therapy.[24]

Because of the difficulty of clinical attribution of causal relationships in pharmacosurveillance, a series of approaches have been proposed.[25, 26] Systems have been designed to be routinely applied to such cases, using algorithms to assist with scientific attribution or, to use the European term, imputation. Such algorithms place various components of the potential causal equation in varying sequence with varying weights. But, in general, all involve an insight into prior probabilities (has the phenomenon been reported in the past?); biological plausibility (is there some theoretical reason why the event might be associated?); sequence (did the event occur after the exposure and within a reasonable time of the exposure?); plausible alternative hypothesis (what else was going on at the time?); rechallenge (does the same agent given a second time associate with the same event?—this is not advisable in the case of anaphylaxis!); and dose duration relationships (is there more of the effect at higher doses?). The problems with such algorithms include: incomplete data, unclear or inconsistently replicable endpoints, and multifactorial situations (sick people often take many drugs, having many other reasons for their complications).

Complicating this attribution dilemma is the competition between clinical attention for the individual and public health attention for the population. In epidemiologic adverse experience monitoring, it is important to discover whether drugs do things and, if so, with what frequency; in clinical pharmcology, it is critical to understand whether a drug did a thing in a person. In the latter, if an agent is causing side effects (e.g., fever) the agent will be discontinued in that patient and, if the symptom is important, never reinstituted. In fact, the person will be "branded" as drug allergic, presumably for a lifetime. In some instances, in which there are many alternative agents, such as anti-inflammatory drugs, this may not matter much. In others, in which excellent agents are few or the patient has already experienced multiple drug intolerances, misbranding an adverse experience may deprive the person of a significant therapeutic advantage. Further, removal of this one therapeutic agent is likely to result in exposure to a different medication with its own side-effect baggage—not to mention recurrence of underlying symptoms in between removal of the one and institution of the other effective therapy. Both clinical pharmacology and pharmacoepidemiology share, however, the need to err on the side of overascertainment—that is, to always to be on the lookout for a possible medication explanation for what's going on in your patient or in the patient population—as medication-induced illness represents preventable illness, with an opportunity by early intervention, to minimize morbidity and, by early warning, to minimize that morbidity in populations.

Misuse of the spontaneous reports database to calculate a "pseudoincidence" rate (numbers of reports in the numerator and numbers of uses in the denominator)—without a keen understanding about the numerous factors that might be operating to bias these indicators—also occurs regularly. After all, while it may not take a "genius" to understand these principles, it probably does take someone sophisticated in epidemiology! Perhaps the most frequently cited example of this phenomenon was a series of hearings occasioned by citizen petitions relating to the relative safety of nonsteroidal anti-inflammatory drugs (NSAIDS) on the basis of frequency of spontaneous reports of GI bleeding (without reference to such biasing factors as to whether the more benign NSAIDS might be prescribed for people with a greater propensity for GI bleeds, not to mention the other epidemiologic nemeses such as secular trend, bandwagon reports, detection bias, and the lot).

The spontaneous voluntary adverse reactions reports system, with all of its complementary monitoring tools, represents the most powerful signal generator conceivable to facilitate early detection of medically important side effects of medications, drawing as it does from the "denominator" of the entire universe of medical treatment. However, because it relies on detection, attribution, and spontaneous voluntary reporting, it is also a flawed signal generator.[27] Misattribution in both directions may result in over- and underreporting; bandwagon effects and biases may result in overreporting for some, but not for others, and clustering of reports in association with, for example, a single published report or a solicitation from a regulatory authority. Artifactual differences in reporting rates derivative of such nonetiologic factors have been reported to reach as much as an order of magnitude. Secular trends conspire to having new drugs better-reported than old, new reactions more interesting than older ones, and, in general, greater reporting from the sector today than in previous years. All of these conspire to restricting the usefulness of spontaneous reporting to signal generation. The epidemiologist who attempts to create a "true rate" from epidemiologic intelligence won't do so a second time. Indeed, much of the work of epidemiologists in the field of pharmacoepidemiology is to help to educate the naive, who use reported cases as a numerator and sales as a denominator and attempt to compare rates of adverse reactions across drugs, formulations, or time. Except under the rarest of circumstances, such comparisons are simply inappropriate. The proper role of epidemiologic intelligence in this field is no different from its role in other fields: to generate hypotheses—signals—that are either strong and unique enough to permit action on their face value (e.g., a cluster of anaphylaxis following use of a new anti-inflammatory drug), or suggestive enough to form the basis for proper epidemiologic study. Ultimately, the only proper source of the definitive, quantitative adverse experience rate is the properly conducted clinical trial or structured epidemiologic study—but that is a subject for a chapter in another book!

PHARMACOEPIDEMIOLOGY: THE WAY FORWARD

Extending What We Now Know

Powerful though the "signal generator" of spontaneous reporting is, its limitations prevent public health protection at the level at which society will increasingly demand. As a result, there is a need to harness new technologies and refine existing ones. A series of efforts were spawned during the 1980s that will doubtless continue during the 1990s: to extend the sources of adverse experience data and, in the process, contribute some much needed clarification. Starting with the clarion call to action in 1980 of the U.S. Joint Commission on Prescription Drug Use (JCPDU), the Melmon Commission[28] issued the dual charge to society to strengthen our spontaneous reports system, the existing epidemiologic intelligence component, and to add the structured epidemiologic study to our standard approach.

Especially noteworthy have been the development and harnessing of large, automated, multipurpose computerized databases envisioned in the

JCPDU Report. In the claims payment files of major third-party reimbursement plans such as Medicaid and Blue Cross or the Saskatchewan Health Plan in Canada, and in the accounting systems of major medical care programs such as the health maintenance organizations, a vast body of automated data has been accumulated in recent years and continues every day to be extended and expanded. Since the mid-1970s, with the automation of claims payment for pharmaceuticals and the automation of pharmacy systems themselves, large sets of data regarding prescriptions in populations have become available. In those billing systems and in several noteworthy HMOs, data regarding all prescriptions may be linked through a patient-identifying number to an individual. Thus, over time, a person's entire pharmaceutical exposure experience can be assembled and stored in the computer. This permits automated patient medication profiling and checks for possible undesirable drug interactions. And, with the proper arrangement, it can also permit linking with automated data from other sources, such as hospital billings in Medicaid or information regarding hospital discharge summaries in an HMO. Thus, the era of record linkage has emerged. Especially powerful as a research tool for both cohort and case-control epidemiologic studies, these databases may also have a role in population monitoring and signal generation. In the large Medicaid database known as COMPASS,[29, 30] initially developed under contract with the Food and Drug Administration and now broadly available as a research tool to university-based pharmacoepidemiologists,[31] over 10 million persons can be monitored for all prescriptions and all major medical events. Creative use of this and other Medicaid databases by academic medical centers has shown great promise.[32, 33] In the province of Saskatchewan, 1 million persons have all pharmaceutical and medical benefits reimbursed by the Saskatchewan Prescription Drug Plan and Hospital Services Plan recorded in a linkable database since 1975 (over 15 million person years.)[34, 35] And in several large HMOs, between 300,000 and over 2 million persons can be followed for all prescription-linked major medical events.[29] Most recently, large medical practices in the United States (e.g., the Harvard Community Health Plan) and the United Kingdom (e.g., Value Added Medical Products [VAMP] System) have employed the automated medical record, capturing large volumes of clinical practice information, including medical events and drug exposures, in potentially analyzable data sets. This poses the possibility in the future of "combing the databases" for possible signals of excesses in the ratio of possible adverse experiences (e.g., hospitalizations) in association with exposure to any and all newly approved medications. With these databases, it is possible to screen all new agents for any occurrence of a series of potentially, theoretically, or commonly associated significant adverse experiences, such as major organ system disease involving liver, kidney, brain, or skin, particularly if the expected rate in the monitored population is very low. A new set of epidemiologic standards and statistical practices will be needed to protect against "mindless data-trolling" and premature alarm over chance associations.

Similar large databases in hospitals with wholly automated hospital pharmacy dispensing and automated hospital discharge data that include all in-hospital procedures and diagnoses permit the same sorts of linkage to ascertain the possible unusual or unexpected occurrence of important medical events[36] among hospitalized patients. These, then, may permit the computer variant of intensive in-patient monitoring, as initiated by the Boston Collaborative Drug Surveillance Program[36, 37] of Prescription Event Monitoring, as initiated by the Drug Safety Research Trust[9] and Case Control Surveillance as initiated by the Slone Epidemiology Unit.[39] But, here too, much work is still needed to harness these resources for such purposes.

Enhancing What We Now Do

In addition, the systems contributing to the existing spontaneous voluntary reactions reports system can always use refinement, exhortation, encouragement, and improvement. For example, the Joint Commission on Accreditation of Healthcare Organizations (JCAHO) has recently revived its interest in a requirement that all hospitals have a drug information/drug safety monitoring system that provides consultation regarding medication-associated illness.[40] We can and must do a better job of harnessing the drug information specialists, a growing body of consulting pharmacists in major hospitals. Being aware of adverse events, they need incentive to report—especially the help of similar drug information groups in the industry.[41]

Finally, we will need to strengthen traditional epidemiologic intelligence—the practice-based spontaneous reporting systems. Efforts are underway to enhance the extent to which such adverse experiences, once detected and addressed at the clinical pharmacology level, may be entered into the pharmacoepidemiologic sphere as surveillance data. The development of pharmacovigilance centers in France is an outstanding case in point, in which, by providing clinical pharmacology consultation to treating physicians, the French have been able to increase materially their adverse experience reporting rates.[42] Networks of community-based pharmacists[43, 44] and hospital-based pharmacists[45] have been established to develop rapid assembly of cohorts to monitor experience and follow-up patient signals. Physicians can do a better job of reporting, too. Recent demonstration projects in Maryland, Maine, Mississippi, and Utah have shown that, with proper education and encouragement, and by making it easier and providing some reporting rewards, physicians can be encouraged to participate in a reporting system, and that the frequency, quality, and usefulness of reports can be increased.

COMPLEMENTING INTELLIGENCE WITH STRUCTURED STUDIES

Understanding the limitations of spontaneous reporting is essential to ensuring the fullest appropriate use of such reports. It is also essential to the development of a proper complementary social effort at epidemiologic structured analytic research, the second half of the "clarion call" of the JCDPU Report of 1980. A major international agenda for the 1990s will be to develop the research capacity to ensure that signals, once generated, can be properly tested by people who know what they are doing, in resources powerful and rapid enough to give public policy answers that can be useful in important decision-making. Here again, the large, automated, multipurpose databases will doubtless play a substantial role. Thus, a proper program of postmarketing surveillance will require a balanced approach that includes both thorough epidemiologic intelligence (employing the principles outlined in this book) and complementary structured epidemiologic studies.

TRANSLATING FINDINGS INTO INSIGHTS

One of the great challenges ahead in this field is helping those involved with medications to better understand the risks and uncertainties so that their decision-making may be improved. Since medicines work by being chemically active in the body, undesired side effects will remain a necessary component of pharmacologic therapy. The target of pharmacosurveillance is not to make risk go away, but rather to recognize it so that those involved may address it. In an extreme example of an individual medication, in the event of the discovery of unanticipated and unacceptably severe risks occurring at a frequency greater than that which is felt to be justified by the benefits of the compound, the individual medication may, in fact, be eliminated from our therapeutic armamentarium. But that won't make risks go away! It will simply substitute the risks of side effects from other drugs that will need to be used in its place, from surgery or other alternative interventions, or from the adverse effects of the incompletely treated disease itself. Indeed, one of the great challenges for the field is the development of better algorithms by which to compare the relative benefit-to-risk ratios across alternative therapeutic interventions.

It is not only risk that will not go away; neither will uncertainty. The lack of clarity regarding the exact nature and frequency of potentially important, but relatively rare, side effects is absolutely unavoidable at the time a new drug is approved. Indeed, as we clamor for better interventions, particularly for life-threatening illness, society will have even earlier new drug approvals and know even less at the time of approval. On balance, this is a very good thing if we really need a new medicine, but need it only as soon as public health protection will permit it. This will put the onus on the postmarketing epidemiologic systems to find unexpected problems.

Further, as more energy is put into extending and improving the spontaneous reports epidemiologic system, it is likely that we will have signals of more important adverse events faster and more clearly. The large, automated, multipurpose databases will give us alternative settings in which to "check" the signal and in which to do more formal epidemiologic study to provide more definitive answers, to ensure scholarly factual underpinnings for important policy making. And as they increase in number and application, the databases will contribute to signal generation as well. But, here again, until a drug is enough used so there are enough exposures in enough databases, rare events simply will not be able to be detected, much less quantitated. There will always be residual uncertainty. Therefore, the second great challenge is to find a way better to quantitate this uncertainty over time, and help those involved in making medication decisions understand not only what we know but also what we don't know, and why.

The substantial challenges for the future simply add to the excitement and complexity of an already exciting and complex field. The proper application of surveillance methodology to the field of pharmaceutics is already making a substantial contribution to the protection of the public's health. The potential for yet greater contributions in years to come make this one of the most rapidly growing and promising partners in the epidemiologic enterprise.

Notes
1. Lenz, W. 1962. Thalidomide and congenital abnormalities. *Lancet* 1:45.
2. Jansen, W. F. 1981. Outline of the history of U.S. drug regulation and labeling. *Food, Drug, Cosmetic Law J* August:420.
3. DiMasi, J. 1990. CSDD Study. *The Pink Sheet* 52(17):April 23. Chevy Chase, Md.: FDC Reports.
4. Idanpaan-Heikkila, J. 1983. *A Review of Safety Information Obtained from Phases I, II, and III Clinical Investigations of Sixteen Selected Drugs*. Rockville, Md.: Food and Drug Administration, Center for Drug and Biologics.

5. Jick, H. 1974. Drugs: remarkably nontoxic. NEJM 291:824–828.
6. Faich, G. A., J. B. Milstien, C. Anello, and C. Baum. 1987. Sources of spontaneous adverse drug reaction reports received by pharmaceutical manufacturers. *Drug Info J* 21:251–255.
7. Milstien, J. B., G. A. Faich, J. P. Hsu, D. E. Knapp, C. Baum, and M. W. Dreis. 1986. Factors affecting physician reporting of adverse drug reactions. *Drug Info J* 20:157–164.
8. Rogers, A. S. 1990. FDA-sponsored project to promote physician reporting of adverse drug events in Maryland 1985–1988. *Clin Res Prac Reg Aff* 8:29.
9. Inman, W. H. W. 1986. *Monitoring for Drug Safety*. 2nd ed., U.K: MTP Press.
10. Mann, R. 1987. *Adverse Drug Reactions*. Lancashire, U.K.: Partheman.
11. Council of Internal Organizations for the Medical Services 1990. *International Reporting of Adverse Drug Reactions*. Geneva: CIOMS.
12. Kono, R. Trends and lessons of SMON research. In Soda, T., ed. 1980. *Drug-Induced Sufferings*, 11. Princeton, N.J.: Excerpta Medica.
13a. Crane, J., N. Pearce, R. Beasley, C. Burgess. Asthma severity and fenoterol prescribing. *New Zealand Medical Journal* 104:147.
13b. Sears, M. and D. R. Taylor. Asthma and beta agonists. *New Zealand Medical Journal* 104:147.
14. World Health Organization. 1988. *Adverse Drug Reactions: A Global Inspection on Signal Generation and Analysis*. Uppsala, Sweden: WHO.
15. U.S. Department of Health and Human Services (USDHHS). 1985. New drug and antibiotic regulations, section 314.80: postmarketing reporting of adverse drug experiences. *Fed Reg* 50(30):7452–7519.
16. U.S. Government Accounting Office. 1990. *FDA Drug Review: Post-approved Risks 1976–1985*. PEMD-90-15. Gaithersburg, Md.: USGAO.
17. Venning, G. R. 1983. Identification of adverse reactions to new drugs. I. What have been the important adverse reactions since thalidomide? *Br Med J* 286:199–202.
18. Venning, G. R. 1983. Identification of adverse reactions to new drugs. II. How were 18 important adverse reactions discovered and with what delays? *Br Med J* 286:289–292.
19. Venning, G. R. 1983. Identification of adverse reactions to new drugs. II. (continued) How were 18 important adverse reactions discovered and with what delays? *Br Med J* 286:365–368.
20. Venning, G. R. 1983. Identification of adverse reactions to new drugs. III. Alerting processes and early warning systems. *Br Med J* 286:458–460.
21. Venning, G. R. 1983. Identification of adverse reactions to new drugs. IV. Verification of suspected adverse reactions. *Br Med J* 286:544–547.
22. Rossi, A. C., L. Bosco, G. A. Faich, A. Tanner, and R. Temple. 1988. The importance of adverse reaction reporting by physicians: Suprofen and the flank pain syndrome. *JAMA* 259:1203–1204.
23. Fagius, J., P. O. Osterman, A. Sidén, and B. E. Wiholm. 1985. Guillain-Barré syndrome following zimelidine treatment. *J Neurol Neurosurg Psychiatry* 48:65–69.

24. Moore, R. D., J. Hidalgo, B. Sugland, and R. Chaisson. 1991. Impact of Zidovudine and other factors of the national history of AIDS. *NEJM* 324:1412–1416.
25. Karch, F. E., and L. Lasagna. 1977. Toward the operational identification of adverse drug reactions. *Clin Pharmacol Ther* 21:247–254.
26. Kramer, M. S., J. M. Leventhal, T. A. Hutchinson, and A. R. Feinstein. 1979. An algorithm for the operational assessment of adverse drug reactions. *JAMA* 242:623–632.
27. Juergens, J. 1990. Controversies in adverse drug reaction reporting. *Am J Hosp Pharm* 47:76–77.
28. Joint Commission on Prescription Drug Use. 1980. *Final Report*. Joint Commission on Prescription Drug Use, Washington, D.C.: JCPDU.
29. Strom, B. L., J. L. Carson, M. L. Morse, and A. A. Leroy. 1985. The computerized online Medicaid analysis and surveillance system: a new resource for post marketing drug surveillance. *Clin Pharmacol Ther* 38:359–364.
30. Strom, B. L., and J. L. Carson. 1989. Automated data bases used for pharmacoepidemiology research. *Clin Pharmacol Thera* 46:390–394.
31. Avorn, J. 1990. Medicaid-based pharmacoepidemiology: claims and contributions. *Epidemiol* 1 & 2:98.
32. Ray, W. A., and M. R. Griffin. 1989. The use of Medicaid data for pharmacoepidemiology. *Am J Epidemiol* 129:837–849.
33. Carson, J. L., B. L. Strom, M. L. Morse, S. L. West, K. A. Soper, P. D. Stolley, and J. K. Jones. 1987. The relative gastrointestinal toxicity of the non-steroidal anti-inflammatory drugs. *Arch Intern Med* 147:1054–1059.
34. West, R. 1988. Saskatchewan Health data bases: a developing resource. Progress in pharmacoepidemiology. *Am J Prev Med* (Suppl)25–27.
35. Downey, W., and L. Strand. Current status of the Saskatchewan Drug Plan. In Edlavitch, S., ed. 1989. *Pharmacoepidemiology: Proceedings of the Third International Conference on Pharmacoepidemiology, Minneapolis, 1987*. Ann Arbor, Mich.: Lewis Publishers.
36. Burke, J. P., H. H. Tilson, and R. Platt. 1989. Expanding roles of hospital epidemiology: pharmacoepidemiology. *Infect Control Hosp Epidemiol* 10:253–254.
37. Jick, H., and O. S. Miettinen. 1976. Regular aspirin use and myocardial infarction. *Br Med J* 1:1057.
38. Miller, R. R., and D. J. Greenblatt. 1976. *Drug Effects in Hospitalized Patients*. New York: John Wiley & Sons.
39. Slone, D., S. Shapiro, and O. S. Miettinen. Case-control surveillance of serious illnesses attributable to ambulatory drug use. In Colombo, F., S. Shapiro, D. Slone, and G. Tognoni, eds. 1977. *Epidemiological Evaluation of Drugs*. Littleton, Mass: PSG Publishing.
40. Joint Commission for Accreditation of Health Care Organizations (JCAHO). 1988. The definition and review of all significant untoward drug reactions. *Accreditation Manual for Hospitals*, 129.
41. Tilson, H., G. E. Collins, and R. Simpson. Post-marketing experience with

drug products. In Pickering, W. R., ed. 1990. *Guides to Information Sources,* 242–262. Bowker-Sour Ltd.
42. Champey, Y., P. S. Lietman, M. Pierredon, and H. Tilson. 1990. *Pharmaco-epidemiology Policy: Practice and Promise.* Proceedings of a symposium sponsored by Foundation Rhone Poulenc Santé, Paris, June 1990.
43. Borden, E. K., and J. G. Lee. 1982. A methodologic study of post-marketing drug evaluation using a pharmacy-based approach. *J Chronic Dis* 35:803–816.
44. Luscombe, F. A. 1985. Methodologic issues in pharmacy-based post-marketing surveillance. *Drug Info J* 19:269–274.
45. Grasela, T. H., Jr., and J. J. Schentag. 1987. A clinical pharmacy-oriented drug surveillance network. I. Program description. *Drug Intell Clin Pharm* 21:902–908.

Index